DISSOCIATION RESOURCE GUIDE

CAROLYN SPRING

THIRD EDITION

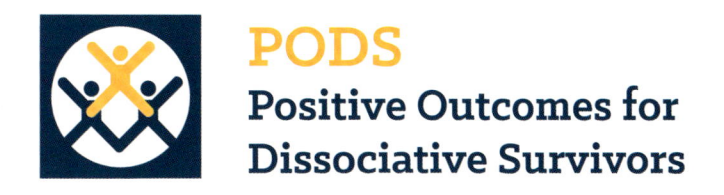

PODS
Positive Outcomes for
Dissociative Survivors

Published by Carolyn Spring Publishing (Huntingdon, UK) on behalf of PODS (Positive Outcomes for Dissociative Survivors).

PODS is a project run by START (Survivors Trauma and Abuse Recovery Trust), a Registered Charity number 1161950.

3 Archers Court, Huntingdon, PE29 6XG, UK

0800 181 4420 (helpline)
01480 413582 (support)
01480 878409 (office)
www.pods-online.org.uk
info@pods-online.org.uk

© 2015 Carolyn Spring.

DSM-5: What's New © 2013 Rob Spring
For Better, For Worse © 2009 Rob Spring
The Problem of Prevalence © 2012 Karen Johnson

Third edition.
First published in 2012.

All content written and collated by Carolyn Spring unless otherwise indicated.

This book is in copyright. No reproduction of any part may take place without the written permission of PODS.

ISBN: 978-0-9929619-0-9

Cover image © Deyan Georgiev - Fotolia.com

Contents

Five 'F' Responses to Trauma	5
What is Psychological Trauma?	6
What is Dissociation?	7
Chronic Dissociation	8
Treatment Approaches	9
What is Dissociative Identity Disorder?	10
What Causes DID?	12
Diagnosis	13
Diagnostic Criteria	15
DSM-5: What's New *Rob Spring*	16
What happened to DDNOS?	20
Medication and DID	21
Diagnostic Tools	22
How Common are Dissociative Disorders?	23
How Common is DID?	24
What Predicts a Poor Outcome in Treating DID?	25
Signs and Symptoms of DID	26
For Better, for Worse *Rob Spring*	28
Parts are Only Part of the Problem	34
Dissociative Moments	40
Pseudogenic, Iatrogenic, Traumagenic?	43
The Problem of Prevalence *Karen Johnson*	50
Book List	54
References	56

PODS (Positive Outcomes for Dissociative Survivors) works to make recovery from dissociative disorders a reality through training, informing and supporting.

PODS provides:
- training days about dissociation, trauma and sexual abuse
- mutual support opportunities for survivors, partners and supporters
- a weekly telephone helpline
- ongoing email support
- resources such as our magazine *Multiple Parts*, Resource Guides and Emergency DID Information Cards
- a register of UK-based 'dissociation-friendly therapists'
- signposting to other organisations.

Please take care when reading as some content may be triggering.

Carolyn Spring carolyn@pods-online.org.uk
Director

Rob Spring rob@pods-online.org.uk
Director

Andy Stephens andy@pods-online.org.uk
Operations Manager

Karen Johnson karen@pods-online.org.uk
Information Manager

Five 'F' Responses to Trauma

As human beings we respond instinctively and from very primitive parts of our brain when faced with overwhelming threat such as trauma. Researchers have identified five innate and automatic responses to threat which dictate much of our behaviour. Understanding this helps to explain why people respond the way they do during abuse and how many people carry these automatic reactions through the rest of life. Many people have heard of the 'fight or flight' response but these are just two of five predictable patterns of responding to threatening situations, all of which can be represented by the letter 'F'. We tend to respond on a sliding scale, depending on how serious the threat.

FRIEND

The first defensive strategy available to us is 'friend'. A newborn baby, who is otherwise immobile and defenceless, has this strategy immediately and can cry for attention and to elicit help. The strategy is to invite a caregiver to come close. After about four to six weeks a baby begins to develop a wider repertoire of eliciting care and attention, including smiling. Later on, with improved motor function, a baby can raise their arms to be picked up and with crawling and walking they can move towards their safe person. So this 'friend' approach (also known as attachment) is based on a small person encouraging contact and protection from a big person. As adults, when in danger we turn to others to help us: if our car has broken down, we may call a partner, a friend or the RAC! (Interestingly this 'social engagement system' is often damaged in abuse survivors and they are either less likely to ask for help or to ask for help excessively, having little confidence in their own abilities to solve a situation or protect themselves.)

FIGHT

The second defensive response, if 'friend' doesn't work, is 'fight'. When threatened, we might respond with overt aggression or more subtle 'fight behaviours' such as saying 'no'.

FLIGHT

The third defensive response is 'flight'. This involves any means of putting distance between the individual and the threat—the most obvious is running away. For both the 'fight' and 'flight' responses, the brain releases a cascade of hormones that provide increased energy to the large muscles. This is the rush of energy associated with anger (a 'fight' response) such as clenched fists and jaw, tension in the shoulders, and the heart-pounding and shakiness we experience when we have just had a near-miss in the car: it is the adrenaline in our bloodstream which was provided in milliseconds to enable us to respond. This all happens before we have had time to consciously think and plan, because it is mediated by very primitive, instinctive parts of our brains.

FREEZE

When the brain perceives that 'friend', 'fight' and 'flight' will not work, it elicits from the body a 'freeze' response. It is thought that the immobility produced by a freeze response has a number of advantages from a survival perspective, including not being detected by a predator. But the body is also flooded with 'homemade heroin', otherwise known as endogenous opioids, and there is a protective numbing of the body and mind in the event of inevitable harm. Being immobile prevents further injury when wounded and allows the body the best chance to survive and recover. The 'freeze' response is exceptionally common in child sexual abuse, as the child's brain automatically perceives that 'friend', 'fight' and 'flight' will not be effective due to the abuser's aggression and superior size and strength. Therefore the brain kicks into a 'freeze' response and the child is literally frozen and paralysed. Unfortunately many abusers take this response to mean consent, and many survivors feel terrible shame for not having fought back or tried to escape. However, they had no choice in the matter as this was literally an automatic body response.

FLOP

If the freeze mechanism fails, the final defensive strategy is employed, which is to 'flop'. This is a state of total submission when all the muscles go floppy and both the body and mind become malleable. 'Higher thinking' processes in the brain are shut off at this point, resulting in a zombie-like submission where people do what they are told and do not protest at all about what is happening to them.

Which 'F' is engaged at any point will depend on a number of factors, principally what is likely to best promote survival and what has been successful or unsuccessful in the past. It is this element of past experience which has a huge bearing on the automatic responses of abuse survivors. Even as adults they are likely to go straight into a 'freeze' or 'flop' response when faced with fairly minor current-day threats (or even just perception of threats) because 'friend', 'fight' and 'flight' were so ineffective for them in the past.

What is Psychological Trauma?

The word 'trauma' carries a range of meanings. In the context of psychology and sexual abuse recovery, it is not simply referring to something very difficult or upsetting. Bessel van der Kolk defines trauma as 'an inescapably stressful event that overwhelms people's existing coping mechanisms' (van der Kolk & Fisler, 1995). A definition offered by Karen Saakvitne is:

'Psychological trauma is the unique individual experience of an event or of enduring conditions in which the individual's ability to integrate his or her emotional experience is overwhelmed (i.e. his or her ability to stay present, understand what is happening, integrate the feelings, and make sense of the experience), or the individual experiences (subjectively) a threat to life, bodily integrity, or sanity'
(Pearlman & Saakvitne, 1995, p. 60).

So trauma is an event or series of events that are so overwhelming and threatening to life or sanity that a person cannot cope. The mind may switch off (dissociate) during the event or, at the very least, it will not be able to hold together the different elements of the event afterwards and 'integrate' them or join them together. For instance, feelings may be separated off from thoughts, or the cognitive understanding of what is happening may be cut off from the sensory experience. It is this lack of 'integration' which characterises trauma. Consequently, the traumatised individual may not be able to think coherently about what happened, or express or connect their feelings about the experience. The traumatic events can be stored 'separately' in the mind from normal, everyday experience and in some cases this will result in actual amnesia.

When the mind is overwhelmed by trauma, it finds it hard to store the event(s) as past memory. For a traumatised individual, the event continues to be experienced as 'present', as 'still happening', because the brain has not been able to integrate the whole experience and mark it with a kind of 'context stamp' that says 'this is over'. It is therefore not surprising that the traumatised person continues to act and feel as if the trauma is still happening, and be over-reactive and hyper-vigilant. In order to cope with this, the traumatised individual may then try to shut off from the 'now' experience of trauma by numbing and avoidance. This then represents the triad of symptoms of PTSD (post-traumatic stress disorder): persistent re-experiencing of the event, avoidance of reminders and numbing of responsiveness, and hyperarousal. PTSD makes perfect sense in the light of the trauma being interpreted as still 'now'.

Many people believe that talking about traumatic events will make things worse. This belief can be part of the 'avoidance' of trauma that people unconsciously employ in order to deal with it. But talking about trauma can be helpful if it is done in a way which allows the thinking 'front brain' to stay online, and to re-tag the memory of the event as 'past'. It is essential that talking about the trauma is not so upsetting and dysregulating that it becomes retraumatising. But if it is sensitively handled, the trauma can subsequently be seen as an event that has happened, rather than continuing to be an event that is still happening now.

When trauma is repeated and particularly overwhelming, the only way of dealing with it may be 'mental flight'. The child distances themselves from what is happening by 'checking out' mentally and pretending that the abuse or trauma is happening to someone else. This feeling of 'de-personalisation' is also common to adult survivors, who report feeling disconnected from the situation, as if it is a scene from a film, rather than their own experience.

This explains why many survivors struggle to feel that anything bad actually happened to them—they fear that they are making it up. It can be very confusing for other people to see survivors claiming that they suffered terrible trauma but not apparently being upset by it. Trauma survivors in fact are likely to suffer from seemingly unrelated symptoms such as physical illness and pain, depression, or ways of coping such as substance abuse or eating disorders.

But if trauma is understood as 'disintegrative', then it is easier to understand these seemingly contradictory responses and connect up the dots between people's behaviours and difficulties and their abusive past.

What is Dissociation?

Dissociation is an entirely normal response to overwhelming trauma.

It is a way of us surviving something that otherwise would be unbearably painful, by narrowing down our consciousness, and failing to 'join up' the different strands of an experience, such as our actions, our memories, our feelings, our thoughts, our sensations and our perceptions.

So we may have only an emotional memory (e.g. terror, disgust, shame) of what happened in a traumatic event, but no 'visual' record ('seeing it' in our mind's eye). Or we may have a vivid mental picture of what happened, but it is disconnected from our feelings, so it is as if it didn't affect us: we feel numb or nothing. The traumatic experience is 'unintegrated' and it takes on a life or identity of its own, separate from our main stream of consciousness. For the rest of our lives, we may have difficulty making a connection between what happened to us and how we felt about it at the time, or its impact on us in terms of how we feel or behave now. We may even struggle to connect with the fact that it happened to us at all.

There are lots of ways to describe dissociation and one of the reasons for the confusion surrounding dissociative disorders is that it can refer both to an experience—when we feel that we are drifting off into a fog, or we switch to another part of our personality—or to the fundamental state and structure of our mind. So to say that we dissociate can refer to something that we do or something that we are.

Here are a number of ways in which dissociation has been described, and some quotes from professionals working in the field:

Dissociation is:

- a fairly common and normal response to trauma
- a creative survival mechanism
- a way of mentally blocking out unbearable thoughts or feelings
- a defence against pain
- an instinctive, biologically-driven reaction
- a splitting-off of mental functions which normally operate together or in tandem
- a normal process which starts out as a defence mechanism to handle trauma, but which over time becomes problematic
- a way of distancing or disconnecting ourselves from the awfulness of trauma
- a failure to integrate or join up information about the environment and our self
- an alteration in consciousness which often feels like being detached or disconnected from the environment or our self
- an automatic and reflexive response based around survival from extreme threat
- a way to cope with irreconcilable conflicts in our mind (such as being abused by someone we love)
- a way of having conflicting emotions by keeping them separate in different parts of our mind
- a way of escaping psychologically when we cannot escape physically
- an automatic response when we are faced with overwhelming emotional or physical pain
- a coping mechanism for surviving overwhelming trauma

- 'a disruption in the usually integrated functions of consciousness, memory, identity, or perception' (APA, 2000, p. 519).
- 'a lifesaving response to overwhelming life experiences' (Haddock, 2001, p. 21)
- 'a partial or complete disruption of the normal integration of a person's psychological functioning' (Dell & O'Neil, 2009, p. xxi)
- 'a partial or complete loss of the normal integration between memories of the past, awareness of identity and immediate sensations, and control of body movements' (ICD-10, WHO, 2010)
- 'a compartmentalisation of experience: elements of a trauma are not integrated into a unitary whole or an integrated sense of self' (Van der Kolk et al, as cited in Dell & O'Neil, 2009, p. 108)
- 'a protective activation of altered states of consciousness in reaction to overwhelming psychological trauma' (Loewenstein, 1996, p. 312)
- 'an unconscious defence mechanism in which a group of mental activities split off from the main stream of consciousness and function as a separate unit' (O'Regan, as cited in Haddock, 2001, p. 11)
- 'its purpose is to take memory or emotion that is directly associated with a trauma and to encapsulate, or separate it, from the conscious self' (Haddock, 2001, p. 11)
- 'mental flight when physical flight is not possible' (Kluft, as cited in Sanderson, 2006, p. 187)
- 'a major failure of integration that interferes with and changes our sense of self and our personality.' (Boon et al, 2011, p. 8)

Chronic Dissociation

Everyone dissociates?

Some researchers believe that everybody experiences dissociation to a degree and that dissociation exists on a continuum, ranging from mild to severe. At the mild end, the mind 'dissociates' unimportant information to concentrate on the task in hand. This is a narrowing of attention to focus only on what is essential. Getting lost in a book is a choice to 'dissociate' away from external distractions. Similarly, 'highway hypnosis' is the name given to the lost-in-thought state that people can fall into when driving a familiar route. They are driving perfectly safely and are ready to respond immediately in an emergency but while 'on auto-pilot' their attention is focused inwardly rather than on the scenery. As a result they may miss their turning or arrive at their destination thinking, 'How did I get here so soon?'

In both of these examples, this is not a response to threat: in fact, it only occurs when the threat-level is low and there is a relative sense of environmental 'safety'. For that reason some researchers do not think that this is the same kind of dissociation as is caused by trauma and which can lead to dissociative disorders. But many people do see it as existing on the same continuum as more problematic forms of dissociation and say that it is therefore a very normal, natural part of the way that our brain is designed to operate. This kind of 'alteration of consciousness', where attention is directed on a specific task and away from other stimuli, can also be practised deliberately, for example in prayer or meditation.

Problematic dissociation

Chronic, problematic, 'pathological' dissociation develops when there is repeated threat or trauma, especially when it starts at a young age and when there is inadequate support or soothing from an attachment figure (usually a parent or primary caregiver).

This kind of trauma-based dissociation is an automatic, biologically-driven mechanism that is usually an involuntary response and which acts as 'mental flight when physical flight is not possible' (Kluft, 1992).

Probably the greatest risk factor for developing a dissociative disorder in adulthood actually comes not from the degree of severity of the trauma, but from having a 'disorganised attachment' pattern. This comes from being cared for in infanthood by a caregiver who is persistently 'frightened' or 'frightening' (Main & Hesse, 1996).

Factors which make chronic dissociation more likely

Childhood trauma does not automatically lead to a dissociative disorder. The greatest resilience factor is a secure attachment pattern. According to Christiane Sanderson (2006, p. 185), factors which increase the risk of developing a dissociative disorder include:

- The severity of the abuse.
- The degree of coercion and pain.
- The younger the child at the onset of abuse.
- The longer the abuse goes on for.
- Abuse by an attachment figure—betrayal trauma ('The need to reconcile the impossible: that the parent is both frightening and nurturing, both monster and rescuer.').
- The presence of alternative realities (for example, nightly abuse versus daily normality).
- Social isolation during the abuse (no attachment figure with whom to process the experience, so it remains dissociated).
- Society's taboo on speaking about the abuse ('The child almost needs to push the experience outside of his consciousness in order to ensure that the CSA is not verbalised to others.').
- Reality-distorting statements from the abuser (such as 'That didn't happen; you were dreaming.').

How do dissociative disorders develop?

Dissociative disorders develop as a result of using dissociation as a survival strategy repeatedly during childhood.

It is as if a 'groove' or 'track' in the mind is formed—in other words, certain neural networks are strengthened, and the mind develops with a propensity for dissociation as a coping mechanism for all kinds of stress, not just traumatic stress. Using dissociation repeatedly means that a child is unlikely to develop alternative coping strategies. This therefore affects their emotional and their personality development.

The nature of dissociative identity disorder is that the trauma is hidden from view, 'dissociated' behind usually quite strong amnesic barriers in the mind. For this reason people can be well into middle or even late adulthood before these protective barriers disintegrate and clear evidence of a dissociative disorder is manifest.

Treatment Approaches

The treatment of choice for dissociative identity disorder is long-term, one-to-one, relational-based psychotherapy. In most cases, therapy will be at least once weekly but this would depend on a number of factors, such as level of support, functioning and motivation. Longer sessions (75–90 minutes, or in some cases longer) are often required, and therapy may extend typically to five or more years. There is no 'quick-fix' and many clinicians advise against any kind of residential setting, as staying connected and involved with 'normal' life is essential for real recovery.

There is growing evidence that the appropriate therapy for DID does yield positive results. There is a large international study currently taking place which is following nearly 300 therapists from around the world along with their dissociative patients (Brand et al, 2009a). The data so far suggests that appropriate treatment leads to fewer dissociative, post-traumatic stress and general psychiatric symptoms; better adaptive functioning; more likelihood of patients being engaged in volunteer work or study; and less likelihood of them being hospitalised.

The expert consensus is that phase-oriented treatment is most effective. Three stages most commonly used are:

- Establishing safety, stabilisation and symptom reduction.
- Working through and integrating traumatic memories.
- Integration and rehabilitation.

In reality, there is unlikely to be a linear progression through these three stages: the work will spiral through each phase, with a frequent need to return to stabilisation work during the middle and later stages. As well as addressing dissociative symptoms, and working through and integrating the underlying trauma, a third area of treatment is that of 'attachment', with the vast majority of DID clients presenting with disorganised attachment patterns.

Phase One focuses on establishing safety and stabilisation and on reducing symptoms. People with dissociative disorders often enter therapy in a very dysregulated, chaotic state and it is important to bring some balance and safety back to their lives before working on traumatic material. The focus during Phase One work is on:

- establishing a therapeutic alliance
- educating patients about their diagnosis and symptoms
- explaining the process of treatment.

The goals of Phase One work include:

- maintaining personal safety
- controlling symptoms
- modulating affect (managing emotions)
- building stress tolerance
- enhancing basic life functioning
- building or improving relational capacities.

The ISSTD Guidelines (2011) stress the importance of establishing a sound treatment frame during Phase One work so that there is sufficient stability to be able to manage the later, more challenging work of confronting and integrating traumatic memories.

Phase Two work is by its very nature difficult: for many years, traumatic memories have been 'dissociated', i.e. cut off from conscious awareness, and bringing them back into consciousness in order to integrate them into an autobiographical life narrative can be harrowing. As Kluft warns: 'The patient often experiences therapy as a guided tour of his or her personal hell without anaesthesia. When a therapist fails to pace the treatment to the tolerance of the patient, the patient may become overwhelmed over and over' (Kluft, as cited in Chu, 2011, p. 212). It is important to focus again on safety and stabilisation whenever this occurs: DID therapy should not destroy the person in the process.

The quality of the relationship between therapist and client is the best predictor of therapeutic success, and so a warm, empathic, consistent, engaged therapist who is willing to be flexible and work long-term with extremely distressing material is essential. Specialist supervision from someone experienced in working with dissociative disorders is advised, as is avoiding isolation by being part of supportive professional groups working in this field.

A variety of adjunctive therapies or techniques can be used alongside traditional talking therapies, including cognitive behavioural therapy (CBT), dialectical behaviour therapy (DBT), eye movement desensitisation and reprocessing (EMDR), and sensorimotor psychotherapy, amongst others. Some of these, such as EMDR, need to be modified in order to be safely used with dissociative clients. Many people in the field of dissociative disorders highly recommend sensorimotor psychotherapy: go to www.sensorimotorpsychotherapy.org for more information. James Chu quotes Dr David Caul who once observed, 'Therapists should always remember that good basic psychotherapy is the first order of treatment regardless of any specific diagnosis.' (Chu, 2011, p. 227).

What is Dissociative Identity Disorder?

Dissociative identity disorder (DID) is neither a personality disorder nor a psychosis. Neither is it the same as schizophrenia, with which it is often mistaken.

DID is simply a creative survival mechanism for coping with overwhelming and chronic childhood trauma.

The now obsolete name of multiple personality disorder was misleading, as it suggested that in DID the person has multiple personalities, as if several different people are living in the same body. This may be what it subjectively feels like to many people with DID, but it is not the objective truth. Rather, the personality of the one person is comprised of many parts 'that are not yet functioning together in a smooth, coordinated and flexible way' (Boon et al, 2011): the one, single person does not have a unitary, single sense of self, but perceives themselves to be multiple. They may also be experienced by others as such, with different 'parts' becoming at times quite autonomous and identifying themselves with different names. The 'parts' that make up the whole that is a person with DID may perceive themselves to be of different ages or different genders, and will have in subtle or obvious ways very different ways of perceiving and relating to the world around them. It is therefore easy to see why DID is thought of in terms of 'multiple personality', but a more accurate rendering is that the person with DID has multiple parts of a single personality, even if it often doesn't feel this way.

DID is almost exclusively caused by repeated childhood trauma in the absence of appropriate parental support (see Causes on Page 12) and is a way of coping with that trauma, rather than being a lifestyle choice or simply a variation of 'normal' experience. The personality is experienced in a disconnected way via separate 'parts' or 'alters' because of conflicts between parts, and a failure in psychological development to 'integrate' or join together the different facets of personality, memory, identity, behaviour and feelings.

Most people achieve a unitary sense of self in the course of normal psychological development, so that as an adult they are aware that they are the same person they were as a child, the same person they are now looking back on being a child, and the same person who exists in all the different roles in life, such as parent, partner, work colleague, friend and family member. Most people can 'shift gears' between these different parts of their personality without thinking about it, and retain a single sense of themselves and their identity whilst operating in these different roles. They do not lose a clear sense of 'I' either across their different roles in life, or across the lifespan. But someone with DID may find this much more difficult—they may not have a sense of a thread running between all the different parts of their experience, a single, core sense of 'I'. Furthermore they may experience intense conflict between different 'parts of the personality' and may experience some degree of amnesia or lack of conscious awareness when 'switching' to a different part of themselves.

It is important to realise that the different parts of the personality in DID usually exist because of this conflict and because of the unbearable intensity of their feelings. A large part of recovery from DID involves resolving these conflicts so that there is no longer any need to remain separate, with knowledge and emotions partitioned off in discrete sections of the mind. This is the essence of 'integration'—bringing together parts of the self that have become and remain separate.

Although everyone with DID is unique, often they share certain characteristics with others with DID, and this is especially true in terms of the way that the different parts of the personality are structured. This concept of conflict can be seen at a fundamental level in terms of two main types of parts within a person's internal 'architecture'. There are usually parts who try very hard just to get on with normal life, who want to be seen as normal, participate in family and work life, and do not want to be identified either as mentally ill or as having a history of trauma or abuse. This conflicts hugely with other parts of the personality whose main function or role has been to try to protect the person from the kinds of abuse or trauma that they suffered as a child.

Whilst parts of the personality that do normal life often have little or no memory or acceptance of having been abused as children, trauma-orientated parts tend to be overly focused on what happened and can at times be consumed with both their feelings about it and their sometimes frantic attempts to prevent it from happening again: to them it can feel as if the abuse is on-going despite in most (but not all) cases having ceased many years previously. There is a fundamental struggle for these parts to be able to differentiate between past and present. As a result, they can be hypervigilant to threat, wary and mistrustful in relationships, and find it difficult to relax and even sleep: they are on constant high alert. Their behaviours make perfect sense in the light of the kinds of things that happened to them as children—usually extensive and repeated abuse of an often extreme nature—but without clear consciousness of that trauma history, it rarely makes any sense to the 'adult' parts of the person. These parts are just trying to carry on with life and their survival strategy has been to keep knowledge and awareness of the abuse out of mind, along with the feelings that go with it. Often this strategy is so successful that they have either partial or total amnesia of their abuse. It is therefore highly confusing and distressing when the forgotten trauma 'intrudes' into consciousness in the form of flashbacks, 'body memories' and triggers: it simply feels as if they are going 'mad'. It is often only when these intrusions become unbearable—when they thwart the strategy of avoiding and getting on with life—that people seek help and begin to accept that they may have a traumatic history and a dissociative mind.

This basic conflict between two different types of 'alter' or 'parts of the personality' is described in a theory of the development of dissociative disorders called 'structural dissociation', developed by Onno van der Hart, Ellert Nijenhuis and Kathy Steele and expounded in their book The Haunted Self (2006). They refer to two main types of 'alter' or 'parts of the personality' in dissociative disorders: ANPs (Apparently Normal Personalities) and EPs (Emotional Personalities). ANPs are avoidant of trauma and often phobic of relationships and emotions, whilst the EPs are stuck in so-called 'trauma time' with the abuse they suffered as a child repeating as if on a permanent loop in their minds: it has never been fully acknowledged, thought about, and integrated into the whole of their personality.

Suzette Boon describes dissociation as 'a kind of parallel owning and disowning of experience. While one part of you owns an experience, another part of you does not. Thus, people with dissociative disorders do not feel integrated and instead feel fragmented because they have memories, thoughts, feelings, behaviours and so forth that they experience as uncharacteristic and foreign, as though these do not belong to themselves.' (Boon et al, 2011)

This is what often characterises DID: a simultaneous owning and disowning of the trauma, constant struggles with denial, and a corresponding confusion in identity.

DID can often be bewildering to both the person who has it and to people around them. It does at times present dramatically, with switches between parts of the personality being very obvious and quite disconcerting, especially to people who do not understand the reasons for it or the way in which the dissociative mind is structured. However, Richard Kluft emphasises that dramatic presentations of DID are the exception rather than the rule. He argues that 'only 6% make their DID obvious on an ongoing basis' (Kluft, 2009, p. 600). Elizabeth Howell similarly refers to DID as 'a disorder of hiddenness' (Howell, 2011, p. 148) and there is growing consensus that the representation of DID in media portrayals such as Sybil is a caricature that is not based on the real experiences of the majority of people with DID. Most in fact do their best to hide their symptoms, in accordance with the function of the 'apparently normal' (ANP) parts of themselves, which is to avoid reminders of the trauma, as well as other parts of the personality. In a society in which there still remains huge stigma and discrimination for having any form of mental illness, overtly demonstrating the dissociative parts of one's personality is arguably 'maladaptive' as it often leads to rejection, shame and mockery.

People with DID exist on a huge spectrum. Some are able, at least most of the time, to maintain both a family and work life and may even do so brilliantly. Others are severely disabled by their condition and in the absence of adequate treatment have little or no control over the trauma-based (EP) parts of their personality and their switching between these parts. One of the enduring legacies of childhood trauma and abuse is difficulties in managing feelings (affect regulation) and given the insistent, pervasive nature of intrusive dissociative symptoms such as flashbacks, as well as difficulties with sleep, it is hardly surprising that daily life can be extremely difficult for someone with DID.

There is however a very positive prognosis for people with DID. With the right treatment—generally held to be long-term, individual, outpatient-based, phase-oriented psychotherapy (please see Treatment Approaches on Page 9)—there is a very good outlook for at least partial recovery. The main work of therapy is to increase co-operation and decrease conflict between the various dissociative parts of the personality, to work through the underlying trauma so that it no longer intrudes into consciousness from dissociated parts of the mind, and to foster secure attachment through the therapeutic alliance. The main difficulties for people with DID are accessing appropriate treatment that will be stable, consistent and sufficiently long-term, especially when dependent on NHS provision.

What Causes DID?

For dissociative identity disorder to develop, there is usually chronic early childhood trauma along with significant problems in the child-parent relationship. DID does not occur in a vacuum: it does not result from a chemical imbalance in the brain and it is not caused by faulty genes. There may be biological, social or environmental factors that increase people's vulnerability to developing a dissociative disorder. But more than anything, DID develops as a result of trauma and disorganised attachment.

RISK FACTORS

Some researchers propose that there are three factors which might increase the likelihood of someone developing a dissociative disorder:

- Biologically, some people may have a greater tendency to dissociate, or they may have organic problems in the brain which makes it harder for them to integrate (or associate, as opposed to dissociate) their experiences.

- Young children's brains are less mature than adults and they are more susceptible to develop a dissociative personality because their sense of self and their personality are not very cohesive—they are still developing. They are less able than adults to cope with and integrate traumatic experiences. So the younger a person is when they experience trauma, the more likely they are to develop a dissociative disorder.

- Children who lack emotional and social support are more likely to develop trauma-related dissociative disorders. If they are growing up in a toxic or neglectful family environment where they are not supported to cope with difficult feelings and situations, they are more likely to use dissociation as a way of dealing with trauma. It is less likely that they will be able to 'integrate' it into their autobiographical narrative (the story of their life), if they have neither the words to talk about it, nor anyone who is willing to listen and to care for them in it. Traumatic events are therefore likely to remain 'out of mind', or in other words dissociated.

TWO PRINCIPLE PATHWAYS

According to research, there are two main factors which lead to a dissociative disorder: trauma, and disorganised attachment.

But DID seems to develop only as a result of *childhood* trauma. Often the symptoms of a dissociative disorder do not become apparent until adulthood, but it is generally felt that trauma which occurs solely in adulthood will not result in a dissociative disorder. It may well result in post-traumatic stress disorder (PTSD), but DID is a developmental disorder as well as a post-traumatic one. Some people argue that for DID to develop, the trauma needs to be chronic (i.e. it happens a lot) and it needs to have begun by the age of eight years old, and probably even younger. One of the reasons for this is that DID is intimately associated with attachment, and attachment patterns are being formed especially in the first three years, providing a template for the rest of life.

Richard Kluft (as cited by Chu, 2011) offered a theory of the development of DID based on:

- The capacity for dissociation.
- Precipitating traumatic experiences that overwhelm the child's non-dissociative coping capacity.
- Specific psychological structuring of the DID alternate personalities.
- Perpetuating factors such as lack of soothing and restorative experiences, which necessitate individuals to find their own ways of moderating distress.

Elizabeth Howell (2011, p. xvii) says: 'DID is usually the outcome of chronic and severe childhood trauma, which can include physical and sexual abuse, extreme and recurrent terror, repeated medical trauma, and extreme neglect.' However, it is important to note that the overwhelming trauma for a child may not be deliberate and malicious. She also notes, 'Parental illness, depression, or problematic attachment styles may be psychically overwhelming and lead to disorganised attachment. In addition, medical trauma may be dissociogenic. For example, some dissociative patients have reported histories of chronic medical problems and hospitalisations that involved severe pain and unavoidable separations from well-meaning parents.'

So DID is not always caused by intentional and malicious abuse, but on the vast majority of occasions it is. One team of researchers (Brand, Classen, Lanius et al, 2009a) found that amongst their patients with dissociative disorders, 86% reported a history of sexual abuse and 79% a history of physical abuse. A further 94% reported emotional abuse. It is possible that the true percentages are even higher than this, because amnesia for trauma is one of the main symptoms and indeed diagnostic criteria for DID: many more might have reported abuse had they been able to recall it.

Diagnosis

Being diagnosed as having a dissociative disorder is by no means simple. The ISSTD Guidelines for Treating DID in Adults (2011) give four reasons for these difficulties:

- A lack of education amongst clinicians about dissociation, dissociative disorders and trauma.

- Most clinicians wrongly believe that DID is 'a rare disorder, with a florid, dramatic presentation' (p.117).

- The standard diagnostic tools and mental status examinations that most clinicians have been taught to use during professional training do not include questions about dissociation, post-traumatic symptoms or a history of trauma.

- Having received little or no training in dissociative disorders, many clinicians have difficulty recognising the signs and symptoms.

The ISSTD assert that assessment for dissociation should be part of every diagnostic interview, given that dissociative disorders are 'at least as common, if not more common, than many other psychiatric disorders that are routinely considered in psychiatric evaluations' (p.124). A number of diagnostic tools have become available in recent years to assist with screening and diagnosis of dissociative disorders, and a summary of the most well-known of these can be found on Page 22.

The 'gold standard' is generally considered to be the SCID-D-R developed by Marlene Steinberg (1994), which is due to be updated to reflect recent criteria changes.

A diagnosis of DID is dependent on the criteria in the DSM-5 (Diagnostic and Statistical Manual, fifth edition) which is published by the American Psychological Association and mainly used in the United States and Canada. The UK and parts of Europe often employ the ICD-10 (International Classification of Diseases, tenth edition), which still talks only about 'multiple personality disorder'.

Both manuals view dissociative disorders a little differently. The DSM understands dissociative disorders as being chronic, long-term conditions that are developmental in nature—in other words, they develop over a period of time in response to trauma and attachment difficulties as a child's brain grows and matures, and they therefore tend to persist over time too as they are more or less 'hard-wired' adaptations. The ICD, however, sees dissociative disorders as being on the whole acute (i.e. short-term), reactive, and transient responses to here-and-now traumatic experiences. Both concepts are part of the truth, an issue acknowledged by the DSM taskforce, and there are attempts underway to merge the conceptualisations of dissociative disorders for the next ICD update.

» Diagnosis

Prior to the updated DSM-5 criteria, diagnosis was largely dependent on the clinician observing a switch between two distinct identity states. Paul Dell (Dell & O'Neil, 2009) amongst others argued convincingly that switching was a fairly infrequent symptom of DID, and only occurred in 15% of diagnostic interviews. The new criteria now allow for discontinuities in sense of self and agency to be self-reported.

DID is often misdiagnosed. Research suggests that people with DID usually spend between 5–12 years in the mental health system before receiving a correct diagnosis (ISSTD, 2011). Part of the reason for this is that people with DID often present to mental health professionals with a range of symptoms, with the specifically dissociative and post-traumatic ones often obscured by a complex mix of depression, panic, somatoform symptoms and eating disorders. Usual misdiagnoses include schizophrenia, schizo-affective disorder, bipolar disorder, borderline personality disorder, epilepsy or pseudo-seizures, eating disorders, and alcohol or drug addiction. The mean age at correct diagnosis is between 28–35 years (Putnam, 1989).

In the UK, getting a diagnosis for DID can be extremely difficult. Many psychiatric teams do not accept the existence of the diagnosis, having been taught that it is controversial and not supported by research. Although this is patently not true, it can often be difficult to shift this mindset, and a diagnosis of borderline personality disorder or complex post-traumatic stress disorder may often be the outcome in these circumstances. There are a number of individuals and organisations who provide private services and diagnostic testing for dissociative disorders—if this is a route you want to consider, please contact PODS to put you in touch with the relevant people.

There are both advantages and disadvantages to receiving a diagnosis of DID. The greatest benefit is receiving appropriate, publically-funded treatment (i.e. in the UK, via the NHS), although this happens only occasionally. It can also be both helpful and reassuring to be able to put a 'name' to the group of symptoms that represent DID. This can guide both the patient's own drive for understanding and acceptance, and can inform the course of therapy. As shame is one of the most debilitating aspects of a dissociative disorder, being able to connect with others with the same diagnosis can help to break that shame and the overwhelming isolation that often goes with it.

The risks associated with diagnosis include difficulty in obtaining life or travel insurance, and discrimination in the workplace (illegal though that may be). A correct diagnosis is rarely a guarantee of appropriate treatment, and in some cases it can mean no treatment at all as the patient is seen as 'too complex'.

Suzette Boon helpfully comments: 'Diagnosis is important, because it provides a map for you and your therapist to follow so that you get proper help…But it is probably more helpful for you to focus on what will aid you in resolving the dissociation that hampers your life, rather than to worry too much about your diagnosis.' (Boon et al, 2011, p.11)

For a fuller discussion on the issues surrounding diagnosis, see Rob Spring's article 'DSM-5: What's New in the Criteria for Dissociative Disorders' on Page 16.

Diagnostic Criteria

Dissociative disorders appear as diagnostic categorisations in both the American-based DSM-5 (Diagnostic and Statistical Manual, version 5) produced by the American Psychological Association (APA, 2013), and the other 'diagnostic bible' used more widely in Europe, the World Health Organisation's ICD-10 (International Classification of Diseases, version 10), (WHO, 2010). The following table shows the criteria in the DSM-5:

Code	Name of disorder	Diagnostic criteria

300.6	Depersonalisation/ Derealisation Disorder	A. The presence of persistent or recurrent experiences of depersonalisation, derealisation or both.
		  1. Depersonalisation: Experiences of unreality, detachment, or being an outside observer with respect to one's thoughts, feelings, sensations, body, or actions (e.g. perceptual alterations, distorted sense of time, unreal or absent self, emotional and/or physical numbing.)
		  2. Derealisation: Experiences of unreality or detachment with respect to surroundings (e.g. individuals or objects are experienced as unreal, dreamlike, foggy, lifeless, or visually distorted.)
		B. During the depersonalisation or derealisation experiences, reality testing remains intact.
		C. The disturbance is not attributable to the physiological effects of a substance (e.g. a drug of abuse, medication) or other medical condition (e.g. seizures).
		D. The disturbance is not better explained by another mental disorder.

300.12 (DA without DF) 300.13 (DA with DF)	Dissociative Amnesia (DA) with or without Dissociative Fugue (DF)	A. An inability to recall important autobiographical information, usually of a traumatic or stressful nature, that is inconsistent with ordinary forgetting. Note: Dissociative Amnesia most often consists of localised or selective amnesia for a specific event or events; or generalised amnesia for identity and life history. B. The symptoms cause clinically significant distress or impairment in social, occupational, or other important areas of functioning. C. The disturbance is not attributable to the physiological effects of a substance. D. The disturbance is not better explained by dissociative identity disorder. 1. Specify if: With Dissociative Fugue: Apparently purposeful travel or bewildered wandering that is associated with amnesia with Dissociative Fugue.
300.14	Dissociative Identity Disorder	A. Disruption of identity characterised by two or more distinct personality states, which may be described in some cultures as an experience of possession. The disruption in identity involves marked discontinuity in sense of self and sense of agency, accompanied by related alterations in affect, behaviour, consciousness, memory, perception, cognition, and/or sensory-motor functioning. These signs and symptoms may be observed by others or reported by the individual. B. Recurrent gaps in the recall of everyday events, important personal information, and/or traumatic events that are inconsistent with ordinary forgetting. C. The symptoms cause clinically significant distress or impairment in social, occupational, or other important areas of functioning. D. The disturbance is not a normal part of a broadly accepted cultural or religious practice. Note: In children, the symptoms are not better explained by imaginary playmates or other fantasy play. E. The symptoms are not attributable to the physiological effects of a substance (e.g. blackouts or chaotic behaviour during alcohol intoxication or other medical condition, e.g. complex partial seizures.)

DSM-5: What's New
in the Criteria for Dissociative Disorders

by Rob Spring

Very few people with an interest or involvement in mental health can have failed to notice the recent media interest in the publication of the latest update to the American 'psychiatric Bible', the DSM (Diagnostic and Statistical Manual), now in its fifth edition (APA, 2013). It has taken fourteen years to write, weighs in at over 800 pages ('Thick enough to stop a bullet,' as one psychiatrist put it) and costs in the region of £80.

But it has been mired in controversy, with suggestions that the pharmaceutical companies have been too influential in the revision process. For example, 18 out of 27 members of the taskforce who revised the manual had direct links to pharmaceutical companies. Furthermore, there have been accusations that the criteria needed to diagnose some mental health conditions have become too wide, or the thresholds too low, with the effect of 'medicalising' normal reactions. For example, the diagnosis of major depressive disorder (MDD) applies to people who experience persistent low mood, loss of enjoyment and pleasure, and a disruption to everyday activity – which is a reasonable conclusion. But under previous criteria, people who had recently been bereaved were specifically excluded, as all of these symptoms are a normal part of the grief process and not signs of mental illness. But in the DSM-5 this exclusion has been removed, so someone who experiences these normal responses after the death of a spouse could now be diagnosed as mentally ill. As a result, a wide variety of individuals and organisations have accused the updates to the DSM-5 of 'over-medicalisation,' with the possibility that some people will be prescribed drugs when all they really need is to progress through the normal stages of grief and adjust to life after loss.

There has been less controversy in terms of changes to the criteria for dissociative disorders but there are some interesting and significant changes. To understand these revisions, it is important to consider how dissociative disorders (DDs) are diagnosed in the UK and therefore what impact the updates to the DSM-5 will have. Of course, on the whole it would probably be true to say that DDs are often not diagnosed at all! Much has been written in the clinical literature about how often DDs are misdiagnosed—as bipolar disorder, schizophrenia, depression, and borderline personality disorder to name but a few alternatives. The ISSTD guidelines (2011) explain why: 'The difficulties in diagnosing dissociative identity disorder result primarily from lack of education among clinicians about dissociation, dissociative disorders, and the effects of psychological trauma, as well as from clinician bias' and 'most clinicians have been taught (or assume) that DID is a rare disorder with a florid, dramatic presentation' (p.117).

But is this a problem? Many people suffering dissociative distress feel that if they could just get a diagnosis, then everything would be alright. And there are certainly a range of benefits from having a diagnostic label—it can help people make sense in a positive way of what is going on for them, of dissociation as a clever, protective survival mechanism that helped them endure otherwise unbearable trauma. Knowing that they are not 'mad' or 'crazy,' but that their symptoms make sense and are utterly logical in the light of their experiences can be a massive step on the pathway towards recovery. Knowing that the 'problem' is a DD can also help determine the appropriate pathway for treatment and recovery: long-term individual psychotherapy is recommended in the ISSTD Treatment Guidelines, as opposed to harmful and unhelpful treatment with anti-psychotics or a focus merely on symptoms, such as substance abuse or eating disorders.

So getting a diagnosis can be very helpful indeed, although many are disappointed to realise that within the strictures of numerous NHS Primary Care Trusts, it does not in fact lead to appropriate treatment and can for some people actually mean being sidelined as 'too complex.' There can be other downsides too such as difficulty in obtaining life insurance, or discrimination at work.

Diagnosis is certainly not the panacea that many people hope it will be, and in many cases it can actually be unnecessary as a wide range of therapists are less concerned with the 'labels' that their clients come to the therapy room with than they are with the person sat in front of them, whatever form their distress is taking and whatever an 'official' diagnosis or lack of it may say.

In the UK, there are two principal routes towards a DD diagnosis: privately or via the NHS. The private option includes a small number of specialist clinics and self-employed clinicians, and details of some of these can be provided by PODS upon request. Achieving a diagnosis via the NHS is more of a postcode lottery and will generally be carried out by either a clinical psychologist or a psychiatrist. But whether privately or through the NHS, diagnosis involves a qualified professional assessing a client against certain defined criteria, and that is where the DSM, and its European-based counterpart the ICD (International Classification of Diseases) come in. Both of these 'manuals' provide lists of mental health conditions with associated codes for quick reference, and a list of criteria that have to be met for that condition to be diagnosed. Alongside these essential reference guides, a range of other tools have been developed, from screening instruments such as the DES (Dissociative Experiences Scale) and SDQ-20 (Somatoform Dissociation Questionnaire) right up to the 'gold standard' of Marlene Steinberg's SCID-D-R (Structured Clinical Interview for DSM-IV Dissociative Disorders—Revised).

So the basis of diagnosis of all mental health conditions are these two diagnostic manuals and although there is, as would be expected, a certain amount of overlap between the two, they do have their differences. Firstly, the DSM is published by the American Psychological Association and is predominantly used in the United States. The ICD meanwhile is published by the World Health Organisation and is most often used in the UK and other parts of Europe. This is relevant for two reasons: firstly, because most research that has been conducted into DDs, as well as the screening and other tools such as the DES and SCID-D-R, are based on the DSM system; and secondly because the two manuals view DDs quite differently. The DSM understands DDs as being chronic, long-term conditions that are developmental in nature—in other words, they develop over a period time in response to trauma and attachment difficulties as a child's brain grows and matures, and they therefore tend to persist over time too as they are more or less 'hard-wired' adaptations. The ICD, however, sees DDs as being on the whole acute (i.e., short-term), reactive, and transient responses to here-and-now stressors and traumatic experiences. Both concepts of course are part of the truth, an issue acknowledged by the DSM taskforce. But most of what has been written about DDs, especially dissociative identity disorder, is based around the DSM understanding, so even though the DSM is not generally used for diagnosis purposes in the UK, an update to its criteria for DDs does have an impact on many people working in this field and its criteria will inevitably be most often quoted in training and in clinical literature.

So what has changed in this latest update? In brief the DSM-IV criteria stated that DID involves the 'presence of two or more distinct identities or personality states (each with its own relatively enduring pattern of perceiving, relating to, and thinking about the environment and self)'. It further stated that 'at least two of these identities or personality states recurrently take control of the person's behaviour', and that someone with DID would also have an 'inability to recall important personal information that is too extensive to be explained by ordinary forgetfulness' (APA, 2000). The criteria further clarified that this was not due to being drunk or the effect of drugs, and that in children it was not to be confused with fantasy play. So the key elements were two or more parts of the personality along with amnesia for important personal information.

Many researchers, clinicians and commentators have been suggesting for a number of years now that these criteria are inadequate, and the update to DSM-5 was the ideal opportunity for their concerns to be addressed. A working group headed up by David Spiegel and including 'big names' in the field, such as Richard Loewenstein and Paul Dell, wrote a paper, 'Dissociative Disorders in the DSM-5' (2011), presenting their recommendations for the new diagnostic criteria. They identified a number of problems, including the following:

» DSM-5: What's New

- DID is complex and has a range of symptoms or phenomena: the current criteria do not reflect this very well.

- The current criteria emphasise the 'presence of two or more personalities' taking control—in other words switching—and yet switching has been found to happen very infrequently during diagnostic interviews, occurring in less than 15% of people with DID.

- Because people don't 'switch on demand' in diagnostic interviews, too many people end up with the diagnosis of dissociative disorder not otherwise specified subtype 1A rather than the more accurate category of DID. As a result, DDNOS, which should be a 'residual category' catching a small number of atypical cases, actually represents 40% of all diagnosed DDs.

- The criteria do not mention 'experiences of pathological possession', which the researchers consider to be a very common form of DID in other cultures.

These concerns have mostly been responded to in the new criteria, which for DID at least are mostly minor tweaks of the wording rather than a drastic overhaul. Probably the most significant change revolves around the issue of switching, of parts/alters 'taking control'. Although an emphasis on this has been retained for diagnostic purposes, the criteria now allow switching between parts either to be observed by the clinician or to be self-reported by the client. It is expected that this will mean that a large swathe of people previously diagnosed with DDNOS Type 1A will now be reclassified as having DID, which will end what many people have seen as a somewhat arbitrary distinction between the two conditions.

The requirement for amnesia in DID has also been modified slightly. The criteria talk now of 'recurrent gaps in the recall of everyday events, important personal information, and/or traumatic events'. This is quite a dramatic widening of the interpretation of amnesia to account for how varied it can be. Rather than just being unable to recall 'important personal information'—which is vague and yet seems somehow quite tightly defined—the new criteria specifically refer to episodes of so-called 'time loss' in daily life (usually caused by switching to another part) as well as amnesia for traumatic events. It is my personal feeling that this will make it easier for people to get a full diagnosis of DID rather than DDNOS Type 1B, which accounted for people who did not apparently have an 'inability to recall important personal information'. In reality this seemed to correlate to people who had full co-consciousness between their alters/parts, which in my experience at least seems to be far more common than is usually admitted. Therefore people who do not experience ongoing time loss as they switch between parts can still qualify for DID, as I understand it, because of their lack of memory for the traumatic events in early childhood which led to their dissociative disorder in the first place. We will have to wait and see how tools such as the SCID-D-R are updated and how they interpret this criterion, but it seems to me that it will ensure that far more people will be identified as having DID rather than being left in limbo with DDNOS-1 over what is to a large extent a technicality.

As recommended by Spiegel et al (2011), the new DID criteria also includes a reference to 'an experience of possession'. It will be interesting to see how this is interpreted, especially in more evangelical Christian circles, and it is worth reading the original text of Spiegel et al's article to understand their reasons for pushing for this characteristic to be included in the criteria. There are numerous first-hand accounts of dissociative survivors undergoing unhelpful and at times retraumatising 'deliverance' sessions within some evangelical circles, where the presence of parts/alters has been mistaken as demonic possession/oppression. The new criteria will hopefully help to engage Christian ministers in better understanding the effects of trauma.

The final thing to note is that there is a new requirement within the DID criteria for the condition to cause 'clinically significant distress or impairment in social, occupational, or other important areas of functioning' (Criterion C). This brings DID into line with the other DDs where for example in DSM-IV depersonalisation disorder (300.6), dissociative amnesia (300.12) and dissociative fugue (300.13) all carried such a requirement. I have not read any rationale for this but if it is applied rigorously it will exclude from positive diagnosis people who claim that DID is a natural state (rather than a developmental consequence of trauma) and who claim that they 'enjoy' having the condition: for it to be diagnosed, it must cause distress.

Inherent, therefore, in the new criteria for DID are changes that will mean that what has been known up to this point as DDNOS will be far less frequently diagnosed, and it should therefore become what it was intended as—a residual category for a few atypical cases. Whilst this is a positive move, the APA are bound to cause some degree of confusion by changing the name of DDNOS and splitting it into two sister categories: other specified dissociative disorder (OSDD) and unspecified dissociative disorder (UDD). But if the majority of DDNOS-1 cases are reclassified as DID, it may be an astute move as the old category of 'DDNOS' is more or less disbanded and the new OSDD/UDD category applied as intended to only a very few atypical cases.

So what is this new OSDD/UDD diagnosis all about? Quite simply, it is designed to be applied to people who do not meet the full criteria for one of the other DDs. In both cases the DSM-5 says: 'This category applies to presentations in which symptoms characteristic of a dissociative disorder that cause clinically significant distress or impairment in social, occupational, or other important areas of functioning predominate, but do not meet the full criteria for any of the disorders in the dissociative disorder class.' The distinction between the two categories then comes down to whether the clinician wants to expound on why the person has not met the criteria for a specific DD. If they do, for example 'dissociative trance', then the diagnosis is 'other specified dissociative disorder', with the reason added. But when there is not enough information to make a more specific diagnosis, for example in A&E, then the (presumably temporary) diagnosis will be given as 'unspecified dissociative disorder'.

Finally, there is one other significant change to the criteria for DDs although in many ways it is a technicality and of much less relevance to people with DID. This is the fact that dissociative fugue has been dropped as a separate disorder and has been conflated with dissociative amnesia (DA). DA can now be diagnosed either on its own or 'with dissociative fugue'. It was felt that there was not sufficient 'clinical utility' to keep the two categories separate as it affected so few people.

It could be argued that, as the ICD is favoured over the DSM in the UK, these updates in DSM-5 will not really affect many people on a practical level. But I do think that there will be a few direct impacts. Firstly, we await the necessary changes that will have to be made to the diagnostic tool, the SCID-D-R and see how that will affect diagnosis. Secondly, it will be interesting to see how epidemiological research is impacted and whether new prevalence studies show DID as even higher than the 1-3% of the general population that the ISSTD accepts. With the migration of many people currently assessed as having DDNOS-1 into the more inclusive set of criteria for DID, it could be that rates do jump significantly—we will have to wait and see. Thirdly, the transition of language from DDNOS to OSDD and UDD is bound to cause some confusion for probably a number of years. Hopefully this will be mitigated at least in part by people who were previously labelled as DDNOS now having the more realistic diagnosis of DID.

In terms of the criteria for DID, I am sure that there are many people who will remain dissatisfied that they seem to focus so centrally on the phenomenon of switching between parts, even though this can now be self-reported, when there are such a range of experiences significant in living life with DID. Spiegel et al (2011) in their recommendations refer to a core of eight symptoms common to DID: amnesia, self-alteration, first rank symptoms (a range of experiences first developed in the diagnosis of schizophrenia but actually found in many cases to be more prevalent in DID than psychotic disorders), voices, trance, somatoform symptoms, depersonalisation and derealisation. The criteria mention only two of these, but

» DSM-5: What's New

Spiegel et al's article does explain the reasons for this: that identity alteration and amnesia are the only symptoms necessary to diagnose DID. The argument centred around whether the criteria for DID should remain 'monothetic' or become 'polythetic'. Simply put, monothetic criteria require for all criteria to be met. A polythetic approach, on the other hand, requires for some criteria to be met, for example 'three out of the following eight symptoms', such as is found in post-traumatic stress disorder (PTSD) and borderline personality disorder (BPD). The argument is an interesting one but research seems to be clear that a monothetic approach is better—it is easier for clinicians to use and doesn't introduce grey areas. And in the case of DID it was felt that it was unnecessary to introduce other symptoms when at core everyone with DID has the two 'prime' symptoms of identity alteration and amnesia.

Implicit within this approach, however, must be the understanding that the criteria are there to diagnose but they are not there to describe. They help to distinguish one condition from another but they do not describe what it is like to live with that condition. Keeping that distinction clearly in mind helps us to understand why switching between parts is so central to the criteria when it is not always evident or visible in a person with DID in daily life. Certainly the new criteria keep things simple and that can only be a good thing.

For details of the diagnostic criteria in the DSM-5 for dissociative disorders, please see the tables on Page 15.

What Happened to DDNOS?

Dissociative disorder not otherwise specified (DDNOS, 300.15) was the usual diagnosis when a full diagnosis of DID could not be made. It now no longer exists as a diagnostic category and has been replaced by other specified dissociative disorder (OSDD) and unspecified dissociative disorder (UDD).

DSM-5 criteria:

Other specified dissociative disorder (OSDD)

This was formally the DDNOS category. An individual who does not meet the full criteria for one of the other disorders will be given a diagnosis of OSDD. This category applies to presentations in which symptoms characteristic of a dissociative disorder that cause clinically significant distress or impairment in social, occupational, or other important areas of functioning predominate, but do not meet the full criteria for any of the disorders in the dissociative disorder class. The other specified dissociative disorders category is used in situations in which the clinician chooses to communicate the specific reason that the presentation does not meet the criteria for any specific dissociative disorder. This is done by recording 'other specified dissociative disorder' followed by a specific reason (e.g. 'Dissociative Trance'.)

Unspecified dissociative disorder (UDD)

This category applies to presentations in which symptoms characteristic of a dissociative disorder that cause clinically significant distress or impairment in social, occupational, or other important area of functioning predominate but do not meet the full criteria for any of the disorders in the dissociative disorders diagnostic class. The unspecified dissociative disorder category is used in situations in which the clinician chooses not to specify the reason that the criteria are not met for a specific dissociative disorder, and includes presentations for which there is insufficient information to make a more specific diagnosis (e.g. in emergency room settings.)

Medication and DID

This page highlights some issues around medication and DID but should not be construed as medical advice.

Dissociative identity disorder (DID) is a form of complex post-traumatic stress disorder and is not to be confused with schizophrenia or bipolar affective disorder, although it may in some cases be co-morbid with psychotic, mood or anxiety disorders. It may also be comorbid with borderline personality disorder.

There are no NICE guidelines for the treatment of dissociative identity disorder and so the guidelines of choice are those produced by the International Society for the Study of Trauma and Dissociation. The current version is the third revision, published in 2011:

International Society for the Study of Trauma and Dissociation (2011) 'Guidelines for Treating Dissociative Identity Disorder in Adults, Third Revision', *Journal of Trauma & Dissociation*, 12(2): 115-187.

The quotes below are taken from these guidelines, which are available via the PODS website.

Several sections of the Guidelines refer to the pharmacotherapy of DID. In summary they say the following:

- DID patients can report different responses to the same medication when 'alternate identities' or 'alternate personalities' are in executive control of the body. Prescribers should beware of the danger of polypharmacy in this group.

- It is best to keep to an overall medication plan rather than chopping and changing: 'DID patients may have many day-to-day symptom fluctuations that are due to the modulation of dissociative defences as well as their personal predicaments and life stresses. Thus, it is most helpful in changing or adjusting medications to attend to the overall "emotional climate" of the patient's presentation rather than trying to medicate the day-to-day psychological changes in "weather".' (p. 151)

- Medication is not the primary focus of treatment: 'Medications for DID are usually best conceptualised as "shock absorbers" rather than as curative interventions.' (p. 151) Long-term, individual psychotherapy is the treatment of choice for DID.

- Medication can be helpfully used to ameliorate traumatic stress symptoms and comorbidities, rather than the DID itself: 'Pharmacotherapy for dissociative disorder patients typically targets the hyperarousal and intrusive symptoms of PTSD, and comorbid conditions such as affective disorders and obsessive-compulsive symptoms, among others.' (p. 150)

- When DID patients report hearing internal voices, these are usually the voices of their 'alternate personalities'. Unless there is a co-morbid psychotic disorder, these should not be treated with anti-psychotic medication: 'Care must be taken to not confuse psychotic auditory hallucinations with the complex, personified, (mostly) inner voices described by DID patients that represent communications between alternate identities.' (p. 153)

- Neuroleptics are not generally recommended for treating DID: 'Hallucinatory phenomena in DID, even when alternate identities engage in command hallucinations mandating danger to self or others, are usually unaffected by even high-dose neuroleptics…Instead, because of problematic side effects such as somnolence, neuroleptics may lead to decreased function rather than to the disappearance of voices.' (p. 153)

- Sleep problems are best treated where possible without resort to medication: 'Sleep problems in DID are usually best addressed in the overall framework of the treatment, using symptom management strategies for fearful alternate identities, negotiating sleep for nocturnal identities, and using trauma-focused cognitive behavioural strategies to decrease PTSD reactivity at night, along with the judicious use of medications.' (p. 153)

Diagnostic Tools

Used for	Tool	What it measures	Reference	Method
Diagnosis	Structured Clinical Interview for DSM-IV Dissociative Disorders, Revised (SCID-D-R)	A 277-item interview that assesses for amnesia, depersonalisation, derealisation, identity confusion, and identity alteration. Measures presence and severity of symptoms.	Steinberg, 1994, 1994, 1995	Clinician-administered
Diagnosis	Dissociative Disorders Interview Schedule (DDIS)	A 132-item structured interview that assesses the symptoms of the five DSM–IV dissociative disorders, somatisation disorder, borderline personality disorder, and major depressive disorder. The DDIS also assesses substance abuse, Schneiderian first-rank symptoms, trance, childhood abuse, secondary features of dissociative identity disorder, and supernatural/paranormal experiences. Measures presence of symptoms but not severity.	Ross, 1997; Ross et al, 1989, 1990	Clinician-administered
Diagnosis	Multidimensional Inventory of Dissociation (MID)	218-item instrument with 168 dissociation items and 50 validity items. Measures 23 dissociative symptoms and six response sets that serve as validity scales.	Dell, 2006	Self-report (but scored by clinician)
Screening only	Dissociative Experiences Scale (DES)	28-item self-report instrument whose items screen primarily for absorption, imaginative involvement, depersonalisation, derealisation, and amnesia.	Bernstein & Putnam, 1986, 1993	Self-report
Screening only	Dissociation Questionnaire (DIS-Q)	63-item self-report instrument which measures identity confusion and fragmentation, loss of control, amnesia, and absorption. Developed in Belgium and The Netherlands, the DIS-Q is more commonly used by European than North American clinicians and researchers.	Vanderlinden, 1993; Vanderlinden, Van Dyck, Vandereycken, Vertommen, & Verkes, 1993	Self-report
Screening only	Somatoform Dissociation Questionnaire-20 (SDQ-20)	20-item instrument that uses a 5-point Likert scale to measure somatoform dissociation. The SDQ-20 items address tunnel vision, auditory distancing, muscle contractions, psychogenic blindness, difficulty urinating, insensitivity to pain, psychogenic paralysis, non-epileptic seizures, and so on. A shorter version, the SDQ-5, is composed of five items from the SDQ-20.	Nijenhuis, Spinhoven, Van Dyck, Van der Hart, & Vanderlinden, 1996, 1998; Nijenhuis et al, 1999	Self-report

How Common are Dissociative Disorders?

Year	Study Authors	Study Participants	What Kind of Dissociative Disorder	% with DD
2006	Foote et al	Psychiatric samples	Prevalence of dissociative disorders	29.0%
1991	Ross et al	Psychiatric samples in Canada	Prevalence of dissociative disorders	21.0%
2007	Sar, Akyz & Dogan	Community samples: women in a general urban Turkish community	Lifetime prevalence of dissociative disorders	18.3%
1995	Horen, Leichner & Lawson	Psychiatric samples in Canada	Prevalence of DSM-IV dissociative disorders	17.0%
2004	Lipsanen et al	Psychiatric samples in Finland	Prevalence of DSM-IV dissociative disorders	17.0%
1995	Latz, Kramer & Hughes	Psychiatric samples	Prevalence of dissociative disorders	15.0%
1993	Saxe et al	Psychiatric samples in the United States	Prevalence of DSM-IV dissociative disorders	13.0%
2000	Sar, Tutkun, Alyanak, Bakim & Baral	Psychiatric samples in Turkey	Prevalence of DSM-IV dissociative disorders	12.0%
1991	Ross	Community sample: large sample of the general population in Winnipeg	Prevalence of DSM-III dissociative disorders	10.0%
1997	Lussier, Steiner, Grey & Hansen	Psychiatric samples in the United States	Prevalence of DSM-IV dissociative disorders	9.0%
2007	Sar, Akyz & Dogan	Women in a general urban Turkish community	Lifetime prevalence of DDNOS	8.3%
1995	Knudsen et al	Psychiatric samples in Norway	Prevalence of dissociative disorders	8.0%
2002	Abu Madini & Alem	Ethiopian rural community	Prevalence of dissociative disorders	6.3%
1996	Modestin, Ebner, Junghan & Emi	Psychiatric samples in Switzerland	Prevalence of DSM-IV dissociative disorders	5.0%
2006	Johnson, Cohen, Kasen & Brook	Community samples	Prevalence of DDNOS in last year	4.4%
2001	Gast, Rodewald, Nickel & Emrich	Psychiatric samples	Prevalence of dissociative disorders	4.0-8.0%
2006	Waller & Ross	North American individuals	Pathological degrees of dissociative symptoms	3.3%
2001	Gast, Rodewald, Nickel & Emrich	Psychiatric samples	Prevalence of DDNOS	2.6%
2006	Johnson, Cohen, Kasen & Brook	Community samples	Prevalence of dissociative amnesia in last year	1.8%
2001	Gast, Rodewald, Nickel & Emrich	Psychiatric samples	Prevalence of depersonalisation disorder	0.9%
2006	Johnson, Cohen, Kasen & Brook	Community samples	Prevalence of depersonalisation disorder in last year	0.8%

How Common is DID?

Year	Study Authors	Study participants	% with DD
1997	Lussier, Steiner, Grey & Hansen	Psychiatric samples in the United States	7.0%
1995	Horen, Leichner & Lawson	Psychiatric samples in Canada	6.0%
2006	Foote et al	Psychiatric samples	6.0%
1998	Tutken et al	Psychiatric samples	5.4%
1995	Knudsen et al	Psychiatric samples in Norway	5.0%
1998	Tutken et al	Psychiatric samples in Turkey	5.0%
1993	Saxe et al	Psychiatric samples in the United States	4.0%
1995	Latz, Kramer & Hughes	Psychiatric samples	4.0%
1991	Ross et al	Psychiatric samples in Canada	3.0–5.0%
2000	Friedl & Draijer	Psychiatric samples in Holland	2%
2001	Gast, Rodewald, Nickel & Emrich	Psychiatric samples	1-2%
2006	Johnson, Cohen, Kasen & Brook	Community samples	1.5%
2007	Sar, Akyz & Dogan	Community samples: women in a general urban Turkish community	1.1%
1991	Ross	Community samples: large sample of the general population in Winnipeg	1.0%
1998	Rifkin, Ghisalbert, Dimatou, Jin & Sethi	Psychiatric samples	1.0%
1999	Akyuz, Dogan, Sar, Yargic & Tutkun	Community samples	0.4%

Numerous researchers have studied dissociative disorders across various cultures. For more information on research papers relating to trauma and dissociation, please visit the PODS website at www.pods-online.org.uk/research.

What Predicts a Poor Outcome in Treating DID?

Cluster 1—Lack of motivation
- Strong investment in secondary gain from having DID / complex PTSD
- Lack of motivation to lead a normal life
- Lack of development of coping skills

Cluster 2—Serious Axis I Co-morbidity
- Schizophrenia
- Psychotic Disorder
- Bipolar Disorder
- More than one severe Axis I disorder in addition to an Axis II disorder
- Current addiction (substance abuse [alcohol and/or drugs], sexual addiction, addiction to crises, etc.)
- Severe cognitive disorganisation or distortion
- Organic mental disorder

Cluster 3—Serious Axis II Co-morbidity
- Antisocial Personality Disorder
- Paranoid Personality Disorder
- Narcissistic Personality Disorder
- Schizotypal or Schizoid Personality Disorder
- Borderline Personality Disorder

Cluster 4—Lack of healthy relationships
- Current ongoing abusive relationships, including sexual and/or physical abuse
- Current abuse, suicide, murder, or molestation of a family member
- Hindrance of therapy by therapist and/or (mental health care) staff
- Prior treatment with abusive therapist(s)
- History of severe, chronic trauma, especially when ritualised and sadistic
- Frequent crises
- Dishonesty

Cluster 5—Lack of healthy therapeutic relationships
- Severe impaired ability to build a therapeutic relationship
- Poor 'closeness of fit' between patient and therapist
- Severely impaired ability to abide by treatment rules
- Lack of responsibility for own share in therapeutic process
- Inability/diminished ability to handle transference situations
- Little co-operation between therapist and dissociative parts of the personality

Cluster 6—Poor attachment
- Severe attachment problems
- Inability to trust others
- Strongly involved in antisocial behaviour
- Strongly involved in antisocial relationships (including abusing others)
- Lack of empathy (for self or others)
- History of complaints and lawsuits against prior therapists
- History of no positive attachment experiences in general

Cluster 7—Self-destruction
- Severe and persistent self-blame
- Lack of interpersonal skills
- Severe inability to distinguish between past and present
- Frequent uncontrollable re-experiencing of the trauma
- Extreme avoidance of trauma-related material
- Amnesia for ongoing abuse (as victim and/or perpetrator)
- Current or recent traumatising events
- Little or no social support in general
- Patient's current significant others resist patient's attempts to be more independent
- High dependence on mental health care workers between therapy sessions
- Lack of resources as precondition for therapy (e.g. financial, housing)
- Absence of development of personal resources (e.g. friends, career, or religious affiliation)
- Lack of ego strength and ego resources
- Lack of 'psychological energy' due to advanced age, physical disease, stressful events, involvement with legal system, etc.
- Little or no work, school, or other daily employment
- History of lack of basic resources (education, poverty, homelessness)

Cluster 8—Lack of other internal and external resources
- Severe resistance against constructive communication among dissociative parts of the personality
- Undue dominance of child alters in daily life
- Frequent dysfunctional switching
- Poorly functioning dissociative parts of the personality in daily life

Reprinted with kind permission from the lead author. Source:

Baars, E., van der Hart, O., Nijenhuis, E., Chu, J., Glas, G. & Draijer, N. (2011). Predicting Stabilizing Treatment Outcomes for Complex Post-traumatic Stress Disorder and Dissociative Identity Disorder: An Expertise-Based Prognostic Model. *Journal of Trauma & Dissociation*. 12(1): 67-87.

See www.pods-online.org.uk/research.

Signs and Symptoms of DID

'Sometimes I find myself somewhere and I don't know how I got there or where I've been, don't know how I am really, feel unreal, like in a dream. I feel like that now. I don't know who I am that's writing this. I'm not real, whoever I am. I feel like I'm ten different people squashed into one, all collapsed down like a concertina. I don't know where I start and where I end. I don't know where the inside of me is. I don't know if I'm really me or I just think I am. It's the strangest feeling. How can I not know who I am?'

Carolyn Spring 2009

One of the major difficulties of dissociative identity disorder is that it is so often a 'disorder of hiddenness' (Howell, 2011, p.148). Many people with DID have grown up in an abusive family environment where they are sworn to secrecy and where hiding becomes a way of life. In adult life, the stigma and sense of shame around both sexual abuse and mental illness is a strong deterrent to making our history and condition known. And implicit to DID is a disconnection from, or avoidance of, both the trauma and the dissociated parts of our personality.

It is not surprising that many people with DID do not appear to people around them as if they are suffering from any kind of mental health problem. Even spouses and partners can be kept in the dark for many years and it is very common for people with DID to hold down often highly-skilled and responsible jobs where colleagues and employers hold them in high esteem for their professionalism. The need to hide our struggles can be a major part of having DID. A large number of people with DID are private to the point of secrecy about their disorder, as shame is such a central facet. The 'signs and symptoms' of DID can therefore be non-existent to many people.

For some, this seeming normality continues until a particular stressor or life event precipitates a sudden and debilitating breakdown, where the exterior veneer of 'normality' is ripped away and dissociative and post-traumatic symptoms become very evident. Others may struggle at a lower level for many years, holding everything together during the daytime, whilst nights are chaotic and disturbed. Some people are so traumatised and have had so little appropriate treatment that they are long-term, 'revolving-door' patients in the psychiatric system and in some cases require 24-hour care: DID exists on a huge spectrum and whilst the same underlying mechanisms of surviving trauma are at work, they are expressed differently depending on a number of factors including level of support, economic status, other comorbid conditions, physical health, education, temperament and personality.

Someone who has DID may have distinct, coherent identities within themselves that are able to assume control of their behaviour and thought. When they 'switch' to these parts, they may be totally unaware or they may be conscious of themselves acting and talking in a manner different to normal. They may feel that they are just watching what is happening from a distance, incapable of intervening, as if it is not really 'them'. They may or may not be aware of these 'alter personalities', who may present with different names, mannerisms, gender identity, sense of age etc. These 'alters' or 'parts' very often have a different way of perceiving and relating to the world as well as different characteristics, memories, sense of identity, and emotions.

Switching to another part can sometimes be very subtle whilst at other times it is very obvious to an observer: there can be dramatic changes in tone of voice, body posture, use of language and levels of eye contact, to name but a few obvious signs. The person with DID however may not be aware that it is happening at all. They may just have a sense of losing time or incoherence about who they are and what they have been doing. They may pick up the conversation at the exact point at which they left it several minutes previously, before they switched, with only a vague sense of 'missing' something. They may appear to have fazed out temporarily and put it down to tiredness or not concentrating; or they may appear disoriented and confused. For many people with DID, switching unintentionally like this in front of other people is experienced as intensely shameful and often they will do their best to hide it.

In practice, the vast majority of people with DID do not obviously present as if they have 'multiple personalities'. Instead they present for treatment with a number of symptoms. Some of these are dissociative or post-traumatic in nature, such as flashbacks, hearing voices, 'body memories' and so on. But many symptoms may appear to be non-trauma-related, such as depression, substance abuse, eating disorders and anxiety.

Paul Dell (Dell & O'Neil, 2009) argues convincingly that the externally-observable 'signs' of switching between personality states are only a very small part of what DID is like in practice. He says that instead it is characterised by 'highly frequent intrusions into executive functioning and sense of self' (p.227) and that these 'intrusions' occur more frequently than switching, perhaps as much as one hundred times more often.

These 'intrusions' may take a 'positive' or 'negative' form, i.e. they may be 'additions' or 'subtractions'. For instance, a flashback is a sliver of memory that is an 'addition', an extra piece of information entering consciousness; conversely, amnesia is where memory has been taken away or subtracted so that it is no longer conscious. Similarly, an intrusion may be related to sensation, in either its 'addition' or 'subtraction' state: for example, pain that is felt that comes from the past (often called a 'body memory') is an intrusion that is an 'addition', whereas the loss of sensation or even full anaesthesia and being unable to feel a part of the body is that same sensation but as a 'subtraction'.

Dell also argues that dissociation affects every realm of our lives: 'There is no human experience that is immune to invasion by the symptoms of pathological dissociation. Pathological dissociation can (and often does) affect seeing, hearing, smelling, tasting, touching, emoting, wanting, dreaming, intending, expecting, knowing, believing, recognising, remembering, and so on' (p.228).

Dell makes a distinction between 'full dissociation' and 'partial dissociation'. In both states, remnants of dissociated trauma 'intrude' or push through from the unconscious into conscious awareness: these include flashbacks, and the many thoughts, feelings and sensations which suddenly come, unbidden, into our awareness, such as memories, smells, emotions, etc. 'Full dissociation' is when dissociative intrusions are fully excluded from consciousness, so we are not aware of them: they come to one part of the personality, but not another. They are therefore experienced only when a switch to another part of the personality has taken place and there is amnesia for the main 'host' or main part of the personality for what that other part is experiencing, thinking, or feeling.

'Partial dissociation' however involves intrusions that are only partially excluded from consciousness, and involves the person being 'disturbingly…aware of the involuntary, ego-alien intrusions into his or her executive functioning and sense of self' (p.228). Dell argues that the majority of the symptoms of dissociation occur with 'co-consciousness', i.e. with partial awareness, and that the classic portrayal of DID 'is so skewed that it constitutes a serious misrepresentation of the disorder' (p.229).

Dell suggests a list of twenty-nine symptoms which he argues more realistically represent the symptoms of DID. Dell's list is a huge improvement on the stereotyped and minimalistic criteria in diagnostic manuals. He also mentions five 'somatoform symptoms', meaning symptoms related to the body, and other clinicians such as Ellert Nijenhuis stress the fact that somatoform symptoms are just as important as psychological ones in dissociative disorders. For example, people with DID often are physiologically hyperaroused—wound-up physically, with an exaggerated startle reflex, and hence they may find it very difficult to relax and to sleep. There are frequent gastrointestinal problems, chronic medically-unexplained pain, and a high incidence of autoimmune-related disorders such as chronic fatigue syndrome, fibromyalgia and rheumatoid arthritis.

For more information, see 'Dissociative Moments' on page 40.

Dell's List *(Dell & O'Neil, 2009)*

- General memory problems
- Depersonalisation
- Derealisation
- Posttraumatic flashbacks
- Somatoform symptoms
- Trance
- Child voices
- Two or more voices or parts that converse, argue, or struggle
- Persecutory voices that comment harshly, make threats, or command self-destructive acts
- Speech insertion (unintentional or disowned utterances)
- Thought insertion or withdrawal
- Made or intrusive feelings and emotions
- Made or intrusive impulses
- Made or intrusive actions
- Temporary loss of well-rehearsed knowledge or skills
- Disconcerting experiences of self-alteration
- Profound and chronic self-puzzlement
- Time loss
- Coming to
- Fugues
- Being told of disremembered actions
- Finding objects among their possessions
- Finding evidence of one's recent actions

For Better, For Worse
Life as the Partner of a Dissociative Survivor

by Rob Spring

We had been married for four years when suddenly everything changed: my wife 'went mad'.

For four years we had led a relatively normal life. We had been working together for two years as full-time foster carers; we were busy and active members in our local church; and we socialised as much as was possible with five small children in tow. Carolyn had always been very industrious, high-achieving and competent, excelling at everything she did. She was very level-headed, very much in control of herself, and very unfamiliar with emotional outbursts. She was a bit of a visionary, churning out a thousand ideas an hour, but she also usually had the expertise and the drive to turn those ideas into reality. I loved her very much, and life together was good.

So when everything changed, it felt like she had gone insane.

It all happened, literally, overnight. In April 2005 she suddenly had a breakdown. She had a difficult night, waking frequently with nightmares. In the early hours of the morning, I found her sat on the edge of the bed, staring into space, unresponsive, almost catatonic. And then she became upset. She was talking about things that didn't make sense, in half-sentences, incomprehensible and bizarre. She became highly agitated, distressed, inconsolable. And I didn't know what to do. The next morning she awoke with a pounding heart and an unfathomable sense of terror. She felt as if she were locked in a room with a tiger with no possibility of escape. The panic, the distress, the huge waves of feelings that suddenly swamped her—we were both as bewildered as each other. Perhaps it was too many sleepless nights. Perhaps it was a build-up of stress from doing some particularly intense adoption work with our foster children. Perhaps it would just get better in a day or two and we would get 'back to normal'.

We have never got 'back to normal'.

Before long she started to feel that she wasn't in control of her feelings at all. She didn't even feel in control of her consciousness. She would 'lose time', not know where she'd been or what she'd been doing, find herself somewhere but not know how she'd got there, 'wake up' in the middle of a conversation. During the daytime, she mostly managed to hold it together. As if with a flick of a switch, her emotions would turn off when necessary and she would continue to care exceptionally well for our foster kids. She would write reports, give evidence to the Police, attend meetings, go to Court. She would attend training and help deliver training. She would feed a baby and soothe a toddler and read a book to all five of them propped up or crouched around attentively, and everything would look like it was 'back to normal'.

But normal didn't exist on an evening or on a night. By 7.00pm, when all the kids were safely tucked up in bed and fast asleep, she would crash. The professional, caring, competent person that she was by day would disappear, and I would encounter 'dissociation'. I didn't know that that was what it was called and I don't know now if that knowledge then would have helped. There are things you can read about in textbooks, and then there are things that you can experience first-hand. And nothing prepares you for first-hand.

At times Carolyn would seem to just space out and disappear into her head for a little while, like a child engrossed in the telly. Then sometimes she would rock, like a neglected orphan, or for minutes at a time she would fall into a trance-like state as if hypnotised. She would 'come back' again and not know where she'd been. And there was that look—that pained, hurting expression on her face, a terror in her eyes and a stiffness in her muscles—that told me that she wasn't just caught up in a report she was writing. It's hard to look into your wife's eyes and see pain so deep that neither of you can bear to put it into words.

I didn't know that she had 'parts', or 'alters'—dissociated, split-off parts of her personality. All I observed was my wife—my adult wife, this competent woman that I knew intimately and who was my best friend—climbing under the table, in terror, distress and unimaginable pain. Then she would writhe and whimper and cry, and in a childlike voice would say things that would haunt me for years to come: 'I don't like the ropes.' She would gesture with her wrists, where obviously there weren't any ropes now. 'I don't want them to come.' Who's coming? I would think, and I knew that there wasn't a logical explanation to that question now. But I also knew, instinctively, that there once was. 'Don't hurt me.' Don't hurt me? How could my wife, my lover, my best friend, this capable, competent, clever, compassionate woman that I'd pledged to spend my life with, this woman with whom I used to lay in bed on a night and belly-laugh together about some silly word-play or a line from a sitcom—how could this woman now be so fearful of me hurting her? 'It's me, Rob,' I would say, as gently as I could. But she didn't seem to recognise me, and my presence seemed to alarm and terrorise her all the more. That hurt us both.

Her littleness was both confusing and convincing. Here was a little child speaking to me from an adult's body. At other times she would feel cold, so cold, so ridiculously ridiculously cold, and neither blankets nor duvets nor jumpers nor hot water bottles would warm her up. She would feel pain as if being cut with knives. She would feel dizzy and sick. She would feel that there was 'yuk' on her face. She would taste things and smell things and feel things on her skin. And then came visual flashbacks too: of horrific abuse and people and places and things that evoked in her feelings of such absolute terror and helplessness that I knew that something must have happened to her as a child to cause such an abrupt and distinctive change in the woman I knew. When she 'came around' from these episodes, she was disoriented and couldn't remember what had happened, or it was hazy and indistinct. Sometimes I would find her sitting on the stairs, rocking and totally unresponsive. Sometimes I would find her having just self-harmed.

I didn't know what to do. Perhaps typically as a bloke, I wanted to fix it. In my mind, at first at least, this behaviour was 'wrong' and so it just had to stop. Inside I felt panic, fear and anger. I wanted my competent wife back. I didn't want life to be like this. I didn't want this uncertainty and doubt to dominate every minute of every day. I didn't understand what was going on, and I didn't like it. I wanted to feel in control. I wanted to feel that this would all stop. I wanted to get 'back to normal'.

My anger spilled out, at first, at her. The compassion that stirred in me at seeing her so little, so terrified and forlorn, was crowded out at times by my fear. 'Just pull yourself together!' I would half-seethe, half-shout, in desperate, awful exasperation. Looking back, I wonder now how I could have been so callous, but I was bursting from the chronic stress of all those days and nights, one after another, on and on for months then years, of 'madness' and terror and not knowing if I was going to come home to a corpse. I didn't believe in myself, that I had the capacity to cope with this. It felt unreasonable. I hadn't signed up for this—night in, night out of bizarre and extreme behaviour, my wife talking like a child, apparently delusional, apparently 'gone mad'. And then day in, day out, the continuation of our busy, stretched, stressful lives as foster carers to five very small and very needy children. But instead of all the children being tucked up in bed by 7.00PM, that's when the 'other children' came out. It felt like I was looking after kids 24 hours a day. And unlike with the fostering, there was no other adult around to help me. And I didn't know what to do.

So I withdrew. Foolishly, I let a friend come in and take over, and she tried to be our 'rescuer'. I stepped back, relieved that I wasn't alone in it all, but stupidly, mindlessly abdicating my responsibility. It was nearly the death-knell of our relationship. All I was communicating to Carolyn was that I couldn't cope, that I didn't want to know, that I wasn't willing to be there for her, that I didn't want to be anywhere near her when she was being 'mad'. A gulf developed between us and we both fell into the chasm. The 'demon dialogues' began: whose fault was it, who was hurting more, who should solve it, why we didn't like each other anymore. It's a pattern that a lot of couples know, right before they divorce.

And we stepped right up to the edge. We talked about it, we threatened it, we even made a decision. But it's not that we didn't love each other. We just didn't know what else to do.

Things got better and things got worse. I stepped up to the mark. I eventually realised and decided that my marriage was my responsibility, and my wife was my responsibility too. I had to be there for

» For Better, For Worse

her. So we started to heal our attachment breaches, and I'm very glad that we did. Help came a year after the initial breakdown in the form of therapy with a very good although inexperienced counsellor. And our relationship started to change as I forced myself to engage with my wife during her dissociative episodes. I made a conscious and determined effort to commit myself to the woman I loved, even though she seemed to have been hijacked by a dozen or so other 'people'. As therapy progressed over the first few months, the traumatic nature of her childhood started to leak out, bit by painful bit. And then the memories of abuse started to pour forth as a deluge.

But they weren't related by the adult Carolyn that I knew. They were relived and re-experienced by what we eventually called the 'little ones'—the child parts of her that had split off or been created to endure the repeated, overwhelming abuse at the hands of those who should have loved her. These 'little ones' existed as if frozen in time, believing that the abuse was still ongoing, that the ropes were still there, the knife still cutting. They appeared often in the middle of the night, reliving awful physical pain, the 'memory' in the body of the abuse and torture she had suffered. At the time they had had no one to comfort or reassure them; they had had no one to tell about what had happened. And so the trauma remained locked away and unresolved, unformulated in her mind, split off from her daytime consciousness. The only crossover into the daytime Competent Carolyn was increasing physical illness—intense, at times crippling pain with no apparent physical cause, and stifling, continual nausea.

The evenings and nights were simply awful to witness: to watch her pass out repeatedly from pain, with 'little ones' terrified and filled with a tangible dread that 'the nasty people' were going to come and hurt them. Past and present were a bewildering mix. Often she could not bear to be comforted, and relief lay only in self-harm, in cutting and overdoses. These dissociative parts of my wife barely knew me. 'Are you going to hurt us?' they would ask me, and it broke my heart. 'Are you cross?' They found it almost impossible to trust me, even to get their words out, or to breathe. My nightly encounters with these terrified child parts gave me just a glimpse of the sickening atrocities to which they had been subjected. It would take years for the full picture to emerge.

The narrative developed in layers and often corresponded to developmental stages. At first, there were the 'little ones', parts of my wife's personality that were stuck at a pre-school level of affective and cognitive ability. One or two had names—'Diddy' just announced herself as if it was the most natural thing in the world for her to be called that. Others chose names to help distinguish them from the others: 'Frightened' was always, well, frightened. 'Leaf' used to count the leaves to distract from the horror of being raped aged four. 'Good girl' was the description of the one who came always to placate, to be good, to smile for the camera, to charm and elicit love. 'White Bear' was a part referenced by a white teddy bear she had for comfort, which she clutched whilst passing out. 'Ditch Girl' was the one who lay freezing and hurt overnight in the ditch. 'Yellow' was…we never did figure out why she was called 'Yellow'.

Then emerged some parts who presented as slightly older, late primary school, eight years and upwards. 'Charlie' was the fighter who loved Manchester United, fierce and loyal and proud and terror-less. Charlie would beat you up if you tried to nick his football stickers. I would sit on an evening with Charlie and let him tell me obscure facts and stats about his favourite team, while he smoothed a sticker into place in his football album. Here was my 30-something wife huddled over some football memorabilia, talking like an eight-year-old boy, gabbling away about football, reciting information so extensive that it can only ever have been acquired to block out less palatable facts. There were a range of 'boys' in this age-category: 'Boys don't get hurt.' Of course, we know that sadly they do, but that was the magical thinking that they clung to, in order to feel safer. They despised the 'little ones', the girls, for not fighting back. There was a lot of work to do on helping them understand one another, to value each other's preferred survival strategy.

And then there was Switch. I met him one night in the darkness. I woke to see my wife standing near the bed holding a knife. Or rather, Switch was holding a knife. Developmentally on the cusp of adolescence, male but in a sensitive, unassuming way rather than the bullish machismo of Charlie, Switch was anguished and deeply reserved. He felt everything keenly. He felt the emotions that adult Carolyn did not. He felt the rejection, the hostility, the pain. And he had turned to self-harm to cope. Switch was funny, courageous, introverted, daring, and shy. And over time—quite incredibly given his early reticence and obsessive reliance on self-inflicted pain as the only means of soothing and connection—he became the catalyst of Carolyn's therapy, and the hub through which all the parts began to integrate. At first my relationship with him was tenuous, with suspicion on his side, and a tendency to isolate. I felt uncomfortable too. Here was my wife, expressed in the form of a 12-year-old, more male than female, but asexual, easily upset, and highly empathic. Switch was all the emotions of my wife rolled into a tight, dense ball of anguish. It took time to win his trust. But once I did, it was mesmerising. Switch and I watched football together, we watched eight seasons of the mini-series '24' together, we watched a thousand space and astronomy documentaries together. Switch came alive.

And through Switch's ability to connect to me and her therapists, those tenuous, threadbare linkages with Carolyn's multiple selves began to solidify and strengthen. Remarkable work was done in therapy. Remarkable narratives and reconnections were made. Remarkable atrocities were disclosed. Remarkable suffering was described. Here was a panoply of self-states describing and reliving and experiencing and communicating all the dissociated and split-apart aspects of the narrative history that coils together to form 'Carolyn'. Most of it was mediated in some way by Switch. Even the 'big ones', the older, adolescent parts whose self-loathing was spun around a core of childbirth narratives—even they found a way out through Switch. Switch's integrative role was and still is central to Carolyn's healing, and Switch himself was enabled from the inside out, through relationship with me and her therapists, to learn to be.

But encountering in such a manner the extreme and organised abuse of children did not leave me unchanged. I have watched as through therapy the amnesia has slowly dissolved away. An inchoate narrative has formed, and threads have been drawn together from different parts of my wife's personality, her history, her feelings, her mind. Without even supervision to go to, in a strange kind of isolation where there was no-one I could talk to about what I was hearing, I struggled to cope with what emerged. Gang-rape, sadism, murder, torture—these have not been stale concepts from second-hand experience. These have been lived out in front of me, in my lounge and in my bedroom, with a 'little one' terrified at the punishment for spilling a drink, an inordinate terror that is impossible to disbelieve when you see someone you know so well switch to a different part of their personality and literally freeze in terror at something so innocuous.

It has changed my worldview. My sheltered upbringing did not prepare me for the scale of child abuse, the extent of organised abuse, or the big business of so-called 'child pornography'. I did not dream that there is so deep a seam of criminality in our world that exploits children to produce crude, sadistic images of abuse, that people collect these images as if they are stamps, that real, live children are raped and tortured to satisfy a coward's incorrigible and perverted lust. I was staggered by this knowledge.

At times the barrage of mental images conjured up by what I was hearing and seeing had a significant impact on my emotional state, causing high anxiety and sleep problems. Secondary traumatic stress—the way that someone else's trauma can infect your own psyche and mess with your head, just by being around it, just by witnessing it and smelling its stench—assaulted me repeatedly. It was so distressing to watch these alters, these parts that make up the totality of the woman who is my wife, reliving the abuse. And there was no escape from it—it happens at the tea-table, in bed, in the car. Therapists can try at least to partition off their life, seek supervision and find solace in 'normal' life. But this was normal life for me. I got to the point where I couldn't remember what it used to be like, before I knew about this stuff. I got to

» For Better, For Worse

the point where I couldn't remember what it used to be like, when touch was easy and I never knew that respectable people from the middle classes intentionally planned and executed the repeated rapes and torture of infants and children. That sort of knowledge doesn't sit lightly in your head. It's not the kind of thing you can mention to your mates.

When at times we dared to be more open with people, the response was often upsetting. We found that the subject of child abuse, and certainly incest-based organised or ritualised abuse, is a step too far for most. Some listen politely. Some look shocked, verging on stunned. But most ask no questions and few if any ever mention it again. We found the dinner invites drying up, a tense but unspoken distance growing between us and our 'friends'. We had to learn to be wise, judging carefully who we thought would cope with our reality. We sadly realised that denial is a normative response to trauma, even someone else's, and it was easier for people to forget about our struggle than to face the realities of what had so devastated my wife.

I was unprepared at first for the backlash. People politely disappearing from our lives was one thing, but it astonished me to realise that so many people so vehemently deny the existence of dissociative disorders and the reality of extreme and organised abuse. About most things I am a conservative sceptic, but I experienced my wife's dissociation first and understood the label later. So when I began to read descriptions of what I was seeing, it all made perfect sense and it never occurred to me to doubt it. There is something viscerally real about observing for yourself your wife switch to a younger part of herself, relive a traumatic incident through visual and kinaesthetic and somatosensory flashbacks, and experience her lack of connected thinking and feeling and behaving. When I read descriptions of dissociation, like the APA (2000) puts it, of 'a disturbance of the integrative functions of identity, memory, or consciousness, and perception of the environment', then I laugh because it's so real. The definition feels stodgy, like all definitions do, but I know that it describes succinctly the reality I have seen of my wife in her adult-self unable to connect to the memories, the feelings, the knowledge of herself as a child; and then my wife as her child-self unable to draw on the cognitive understanding of the adult, that it's not her fault, that she's safe now, that it's over. That core lack of integration of knowledge and ability, of feelings and identity, of behaviour and meaning, is so evidently what I have seen since Carolyn's breakdown in 2005. And so it puzzles me that there is such a maelstrom of debate in some circles about the reality and existence of DID. Come and spend a month with us, I want to say. Then you might believe it.

Eventually, as enough of a narrative coalesced into words and there was sufficient emotional stability to build a platform from which to progress, we went to the police. It's not within everyone's power to do so. Many times I wish we hadn't. But Carolyn came to a place within herself, not where she needed the external validation of a successful prosecution to reassure her of her reality, but because she was convinced of her narrative: she knew that dangerous people were walking free, and she had no assurance that they weren't still doing to others what they had done to her. The step of reporting to the police in itself shattered our peace: more self-harm, more suicidality, prompted by the powerlessness of a situation in which communication is sparse and decision-making seemingly arbitrary. We had an initially positive experience of the police locally, who were convinced by Carolyn's rambling and disjointed account partly because it was so rambling and disjointed—it had none of the polish of a fabricated or confabulated account. She stuck to what she knew, which at times was frustratingly little—how do you trace a man from thirty years ago who was bald, or a youth with blonde hair, or a house with an upstairs bedroom? But there was enough to begin an investigation, and for the investigation to take sixteen months. The police corroborated dozens of details of Carolyn's story—buildings on farms in the exact layout she had described, places and people and visits and a chronology that was remarkably accurate given the extent of her previous amnesia. But not enough evidence to prosecute, so we were powerless once more.

But the smog that was our lives from 2005 onwards did begin to clear as the pollutants from Carolyn's childhood started to be processed. Gradually, control was restored: nights became for sleeping, days became steadier, more productive, and less volatile. Patterns were re-established of a working week, rhythms during each day. Carolyn continued to have therapy, describing it still as her 'controlled explosion' where the unintegrations of her week are smelted together and given cohesive form. She continued to have DID, but her parts were more collaborative. They began to co-operate, to communicate, to enable Carolyn most of the time to live a productive and fruitful life. Night times could still be shattered by nightmares and pain. Somatic symptoms continued to plague her. She was not healed. That much trauma does not heal easily. But she was recovering. Her life took on meaning and purpose.

If there is one thing that has characterised Carolyn's recovery to date, it has been her determination to 'succeed'. Drummed into her through years of academic and sporting achievement, however out-of-control at times she was, as she picked her way through the wreckage of her posttraumatic and dissociative symptoms, she wasn't going to let it beat her. And she was going to change the world. That had always been our joke, even before the breakdown: we wanted to live our lives to change the world. Maybe not the whole world, but a part of it.

Carolyn's key message in all her writing and speaking is always hope. Sometimes I had to hold that hope for her. Sometimes she had to hold mine for me. At all times Carolyn's therapists held it for both of us. But the fact that our marriage has survived, the fact that Carolyn herself has survived, means that there is hope. Our lives haven't ever got 'back to normal'. But strangely, I prefer the life we now have to the one we had before. I didn't sign up for 'life as the partner of a dissociative survivor'. I didn't think I could cope with that much stress, and that much heartache, and that much pain. But I did and I do. We are walking through this, into our new reality, together. Things will never get 'back to normal'. But my wife is not mad. She's not making it all up. She's not attention-seeking. She's not psychotic. She is none of the things that dissociative survivors are so often accused of. She's just traumatised. And she's recovering.

And most importantly for me, she is still my wife.

Parts are Only Part of the Problem

I have dissociative identity disorder. I have many separate, distinct and unique 'parts' of my personality. My 'parts' or 'alters' collectively add up to the total person that is me. I am the sum of all my parts. They are each a letter, and I am a sentence.

At times, different parts take 'control' of my body, mind and behaviour—this is switching and it can be obvious or subtle. The part who comes out, who takes over, may be known by a different name, may perceive themselves to be a different gender or age, and most usually will view the world very differently to the way that I do.

Confusing? Weird? Fascinating? Well yes and no. Parts are the fundamental, basic building blocks of this phenomenon previously known as Multiple Personality Disorder. People who have never encountered someone's parts sometimes suggest that it's a controversial diagnosis, but the evident reality of DID is unmistakeable and irrefutable once you have. After a little while, it just becomes normal. It stops being confusing, weird and fascinating. And then, and perhaps only then, can you see beyond the label to realise that it is caused by chronic, repeated early life trauma occurring on an existing fault line of disrupted attachment. DID does not develop for no reason.

When you appreciate that DID almost always results from extreme trauma, you can perhaps begin to understand why people do not want to believe that it exists—because they resist acknowledging the causes. It is easier to deny the impacts of childhood abuse than face its reality.

For many years, the diagnostic criteria for DID (for example up to and including DSM-IV) focused on the existence of 'parts' and required visible evidence of switching. But diagnostic criteria do not tell you what it is actually like to live with that condition. DID in my experience is strangely misrepresented: a caricature of it has formed in the public consciousness. Starting with Sybil, the media continues to pursue the more newsworthy, florid representations of DID and to present them as the norm. Typically this is DID with a churlish Kevin-esque thirteen-year-old 'part' suddenly intruding upon the 50-year-old female 'host' (as if she is carrying some parasitic alien) and then disappearing to be replaced by an eager, cutesy six-year-old.

And this media view of DID is something that for some time has been particularly close to my heart. On numerous occasions I have received requests from different TV production companies to participate in a documentary. I discussed one request at length. They wanted to a do a fly-on-the-wall style piece. They were very enthusiastic about it. It would raise awareness, make people understand what DID was all about, bring it into the mainstream. A camera crew would follow me around all day for a whole week. At this point I simply had to interject: 'I'm sorry,' I said, 'but I'm just not that interesting. Mostly all I do is stare at a computer screen, and type. My parts don't come out when I'm working. In fact, mostly nowadays my parts don't come out at all except in therapy, and you're not filming that. I'm really quite dull.'

The producer was suitably disappointed that I was dispelling the myth that everyone with DID lives in an uncontrollable whirlwind of frenetic and very public switching. For those who do, it is dubious whether allowing a TV company to film it would be at all conducive to their mental health. It seems to me perilously close to a 'circus act', being exploited for the entertainment on Channel 4 of the mocking middle classes.

Having parts and switching is fundamental to having DID—no-one doubts that. It is the most bizarre, the most frightening and perhaps the most shameful aspect of the condition, and that is undoubtedly why it garners so much attention and morbid fascination, as well as hostile incredulity from deniers. But I believe that a skewed emphasis on the phenomenon of parts can be detrimental—because there are many other aspects to life with DID. The symptoms of DID are the symptoms of unhealed suffering and that suffering manifests in a variety of ways, not just in the presence of parts.

For me, my initial focus on the multitude of 'parts of my personality', eagerly mapped out in early therapeutic work until we lost count at over 100, has gradually given way to a more panoramic perspective. There are many facets to life with

DID: powerlessness or 'learned helplessness'; difficulties with managing my feelings, also known as 'affect regulation'; relational issues around boundaries and maintaining or even attaining a solid sense of self; the low-hanging, ubiquitous thunderclouds of shame; battles with denial and perception of 'truth'; somatic impacts; difficulties differentiating past from present; and the many other widespread disintegrative impacts of trauma slavered over our entire functioning and personality.

So DID for me is this vast billowy blanket of impacts and consequences that covers every area of my life and is expressed much more extensively than just in conflict and turn-taking between parts. While my switching now is mostly controlled and manageable and even 'logical', I still have a lot of work to do in the many other areas I highlighted above: if only 'parts' were all of the problem…

Indeed, the consensus of experts who wrote the 'Guidelines of Treatment of Dissociative Identity Disorder', published by the ISSTD (2011, p.123), says:

'…therapists who are experienced in the treatment of DID typically pay relatively limited attention to the overt style and presentation of the different alternative identities. Instead they focus on the cognitive, affective, and psychodynamic characteristics embodied by each identity while simultaneously attending to identities collectively as a system of representation, symbolisation and meaning.'

In other words, parts are important, but the biggest clues can come from figuring out what they mean and represent. Why are they 'part' of the whole? How do they fit into that whole? What has caused them to be separate from the whole? What is their role and function in the system as a whole? What is going on here?

In her book *Understanding and Treating Dissociative Identity Disorder*, Elizabeth Howell astutely describes DID as a 'disorder of hiddenness' and comments that according to Richard Kluft 'only about 6% of those with DID exhibit obvious switching in an ongoing way' (2009, p.600).This resonates clearly with me. Only a very few people who know me have ever seen my parts. As I have gained more control over my symptoms, learning to manage my emotions within a 'window of tolerance', learning to ground myself and orient to the here-and-now, learning to anticipate and plan and care for myself, learning to take into account my various needs at the multi-storey levels within myself, switching has become less and less spontaneous and more and more a matter of choice. My therapy session, my 'controlled explosion' as I put it, is the safe place for parts to come out now. It has become an increasingly private affair as I have learned that it is healthy to have boundaries and that privacy is not the same as secrecy, and privacy is okay.

Back in the months of intense struggle from 2005 to 2008, DID was very much a 'disorder of hiddenness' for me, the epitome of shame. I wanted nobody to know. For many of us, the hardest part of living with DID is concealing it so that we are not ostracised or labelled as 'weird'. We fear people's fear, and thus their rejection. Many of us therefore do our best to conceal our parts—the many people I know with DID who work as social workers or nurses or teachers or carers or in business cannot afford to 'let things slip' and it is often that pressure, of keeping everything tightly controlled whilst at work, that causes their greatest difficulties. Few of us believe that employers would really be sympathetic and helpful if they found out that we were a 'Sybil': it is not what we truly are that we always fear, but what people assume that we are, based on myths and caricatures. Managing anxiety is often harder than managing parts.

For many of us, our main symptoms are invisible. The focus on 'parts' eclipses these more subtle struggles: our disordered or chaotic eating; our catastrophic or paranoid thinking; flattened feelings and a chronic sense of emptiness; even the frequent amnesic episodes that we may experience throughout the day—we do our best to hide these, to 'act normal' and to brush over our lapses and blame them on tiredness or inattention or age. We ensure that very few of our symptoms are actually visible to the outside world.

» Parts are only Part of the Problem

DID is a label that can be adaptive because it can enable us to seek appropriate help. That help is only rarely forthcoming through the NHS but, in the private sector at least, knowing what we are dealing with, and having a therapist who knows what they are dealing with, can be a good thing. And the label can come as blessed relief after the chaotic muddle of a breakdown, where behaviour and feelings and reactions make no sense and so therefore reek worryingly of craziness and insanity: understanding that your reactions are normal, that other people act and think and feel the same way as you do, is probably the most liberating, hope-giving aspect of being landed with a label.

But this depends on what the label looks like. If it hints darkly at a lifetime of psychiatric 'revolving door' treatment, a future bleak with wrecked ambitions, failed relationships and weight-gaining medication, then the label gives us very little reassurance or hope. If however we see DID as a condition that is entirely logical and natural and normal—a creative and adaptive response to survive otherwise unendurable trauma—and if we recognise that it is a condition with a very positive prognosis, as per recent research studies (Brand et al, 2009a), then the label can be helpful. If we see others who have made significant progress in their recovery and are leading fulfilling, successful lives, then there can be palpable relief from embracing the label. We do need more 'survivor stories' of recovery to become available in the DID literature to encourage people towards hope and a belief for a better tomorrow.

The label can be adaptive but we can also adapt to the label. Even unconsciously, we can end up figuring out how we're 'supposed' to be with DID. Via social contagion, we can start to take on the traits and characteristics of other people we meet or know with DID and in contravention of clinical advice (for example, again, the ISSTD Guidelines), we can end up with increasingly elaborated and increasingly dissociated parts of our personality. It is a powerful thing to be amongst people who fully accept and understand why you have parts. And sometimes, after living so long in hiding with a suffocating fear of stigma and discrimination, the result can be that we over-compensate and we become more dissociative. For people who would otherwise be strangers, it is all we have in common: unconscious group pressures can end up inviting us to exaggerate our dissociativeness to fit in. Having parts, and displaying parts, can become a kind of membership card by which we prove that we belong to the group. This can redirect us from the safe expression of parts within the privacy of the home or the safety of a therapy session and towards an 'alter-centric' way of relating to others. The label starts to dictate to us.

At other times I have observed the development of a kind of competitiveness among people with dissociative disorders, as exists in every other domain in life. It is not overt or spoken, but a kind of hierarchy based on perceived degrees of traumatisation or dissociation can develop: 'I've got more parts than you', 'I have mind control-based DID, not just 'normal' DID'. I would always argue that our subjective experience of trauma is what counts rather than tally points from some external 'scoring system'; and I would also argue that for many of us the rejection and abuse from our mothers is harder to bear than even the most terrifying of organised or ritualised abuse. Sometimes claims of polyfragmentation and ongoing abuse and victimisation can become a kind of 'badge of honour': it can be an earnest, unconscious demonstration proving that we cannot recover, rather than the tragic reality of overwhelming suffering that will take a lot of hard work and dedication to overcome.

The net result for many people that I talk to is that they end up feeling as if they are not 'proper DID'. Measured objectively against diagnostic criteria, they tick the boxes; even their phenomenological experience extensively matches that of most other people's. But the lingering, murky doubt remains that they are not 'DID enough' compared to others. This is where Richard Kluft's statistic comes in though, where only 6% of people with DID manifest it obviously in an ongoing way. It is therefore logical to assume that if we base our perception of DID on the 6% who shout the loudest (or display their parts the most overtly) then we will be misrepresenting DID, not as the 'disorder of hiddenness' that it really is, but as the cockeyed media representation of The United

States of Tara. So the label can be adaptive, but not if we then adapt to the label and feel that we have to be more 'obviously' DID than we are. By hiding our symptoms, we are actually being consistent with the vast majority, the 94%.

The reality is that parts are just that: an important and fundamental part of having DID but not the whole. We can be dissociative about being dissociative. A helpful analogy for me has been that of having perspective and being able to zoom in and out. When I zoom in, I am right there with one or more of the parts of my personality, for example with Diddy, my 4-year-old little girl part. I am there with the smack-in-the-face reality of her deep longings for love and acceptance, her attachment drives, her magical thinking and desperate need for protection. Or I am there with Charlie, my fierce 8-year-old warrior part, acerbic and feisty with the burden of guilt of forced perpetration. These are very real, very incarnate parts of my personality. They exist, they feel, they think, they want, they hope, they despair. But they are not all of me and they are not the bigger picture.

If I zoom out, there is the whole of me, the me-as-we that comprises every single one of those precious, unique parts. And I can begin then to see that my parts have a function and a meaning. So there is a reason why Diddy is a little girl and aged about 4. She was the one who was able to elicit care and soothing from the people around me—something that I have been more or less incapable of doing. She was the one with her attachment needs still intact, who wanted to love and be loved, devoid of the cynical mistrust and angling-for-rejection of my teenage parts. Diddy was little, vulnerable, loveable, and represented parts of me that I had walled-off and dissociated from, that I could not express as adult-me.

And it was so much more helpful to try to figure out what Diddy was all about, why I needed a Diddy part to be separate from me, to try to discern what it was that I could not bear facing or feeling, than it was for everyone (myself included) to gawp at a thirty-something woman curled up under the desk and speaking in the voice of a child. As I began to acknowledge and recognise Diddy's feelings and thoughts and memories and beliefs as my own, I spontaneously found that I needed less and less to actually 'switch' to Diddy to get those needs met. Instead I became able to tune into what the Diddy parts of me were saying and feeling and wanting, and to respond to that from within my adult self. If I hadn't been able to zoom out from the close-up of Diddy, I wouldn't have been able to place her and relate to her within the context of the whole of me.

But I needed to be able to zoom further out, to beyond myself. Trauma has this terribly narrowing effect of zooming us into the details and we can become almost autistically focused on the micro-message of 'here and now', in the same way that young children can only see and hear and feel from the immediacy of what they are currently experiencing. I needed the 'mindsight', the mentalising ability to go wide-angle and zoom back out to see myself not just as a jumbled and mostly disconnected conglomeration of 'parts' but as a person, unified although still disconnected, and a person who exists in a social setting wider than just me-as-we.

This wider social context exists on a number of different planes: the me as part of me-and-Rob, the me-as-client, the me-as-friend, the me-as-colleague. This is a wider world that involves other people. We certainly don't mean to become selfish and self-centred, and mostly we are mortified to realise that at times we fail spectacularly to empathise with others. Seeing others as a threat when they are just trying to help us, recoiling from their comfort-laden touch, ignoring their tiredness through our own hyperactivity—we don't mean for this to impact them negatively, but often it does. The dominating screech of trauma in our lives renders us partially deaf to others, with regretfully less energy and time and focus and attention for those around us. I had to forgive myself for that, to give myself a break for my 'failures'. But I also had to realise that sometimes I needed to step back from my obsessive attempts to solve the riddle of trauma and dissociation in my life, and actually take into account other people as well.

» Parts are only Part of the Problem

And then, to zoom out even further, there is my place in society. One of my lowest points was in 2008 after I stopped work as a foster carer, which I had loved. Fostering had been a suitable outlet for my ravenous need to overcome evil with good but it is incredibly demanding and in the midst of seemingly unending trauma work in therapy I knew I needed a break. I lapsed into an intensely dark, suicidal phase. After one particularly perilous night, in a particularly perilous week, my therapist suggested that I read Victor Frankl's book Man's Search for Meaning. It amuses me still that a therapist should suggest to a suicidal client that they cheer themselves up by reading an unapologetically gloomy book about the atrocities of the Nazi concentration camps. But it had a profound effect because it zoomed me out to the level of society and made me realise that in my suffering I am not alone. I am not alone. No, and I am not even unique. In the bizarrely wise words of Battlestar Galactica, 'This has all happened before, and it will all happen again.'

I could have stayed zoomed-in just at the micro-level of myself and my parts. I could have stayed zoomed-out just at the level of myself in my therapy and family world. But instead I was being invited to zoom out to the wider context of human suffering, and to see my place in it. I felt insignificantly small. But strangely, this did not make me feel that my suffering was any less, that my suffering was in any way insignificant or did not matter. I was not left with a sense of hierarchy or competition, of 'Victor Frankl's suffering was worse than mine, so why am I complaining…' Instead it left me with a raw, persistent sense that I needed to survive.

I needed to get through this suicidal patch. I needed to weather this epoch of months-becoming-years of therapy. I needed to start functioning again and I needed to be able to do something.

I realised then, in a way that has been etched into my understanding of suffering ever since, that powerlessness is the core essence of trauma and that my battle was not with DID or parts or even the trauma itself. My battle was against powerlessness. I needed to rise up against it, to find meaning in what I was enduring and had endured, and to make something out of it. That story of concentration camp suffering—the unspeakable horror inflicted on human beings by inhuman beings—sparked in me an explosive desire to recover so that I could help to stand against this inhumanity as I saw it everywhere around me: in sexual abuse, in human trafficking, in domestic violence, in exploitative working conditions, in rape, in female genital mutilation, in the lack of running water for three billion people in the world and in countless other ways.

Since then I have zoomed out even more. I began to rediscover the natural world. I began to rediscover the stars in the sky: the billion stars in our galaxy, the billion galaxies each of a billion stars in our Universe—these mind-melting realities of the vastness of space and the minute insignificance (and yet overwhelming significance) of ourselves on this delicate blue-green marble suspended in a void. This was to me a panorama of unimaginable magnitude which became a source of both inspiration and reassurance and which conversely fuelled in me a desire to engage more purposefully at the 'quantum' level of my parts. What it did was remind me that I am just a human being. I am precious and I am valuable, but I am not different or unique. I am not in some discrete category of my own: 'woman with multiple personalities', as if there is the human race, and then beyond that scale there are people with DID. The zoomed-out perspective helped me see that I am normal, I am human, and that there is nothing that has happened to me that has not happened before and that will not happen again. And within all of that, I am not even 'special'.

It is this concept of specialness that began to fascinate me. It is a strange experience to stand up in front of a group to deliver a talk or a training day on the subject of DID and be met with a sense of fascination (sometimes morbid), of curiosity or of bemusement. A thousand questions pour out of a thousand mouths: what is it like to switch, are you aware of doing it, can you control it, why did nobody notice the abuse, how do you feel about your perpetrators, have you always known that you have parts?

And it struck me how many people saw me as being 'different' because I had DID. And I came back, time and again, to a fundamental belief that I hold more firmly today than I ever have done: that I am not special; that I am certainly not a 'circus act' for people to queue up to see, and prod with sticks as they would in the days of Bedlam. And well-meaning though much of the interest in me and my story was, it left me at times feeling uncomfortable and as if it were robbing from me my innate, 'normal' humanity.

I have come to believe with fervent passion that the focus on multiple personalities is missing the point. DID is not rare; it is not unique; it is not special. It is just a logical set of symptoms to some terrible trauma. It is a normal way to react to very abnormal childhood treatment. In fact, I only have DID because I am normal. If I had not reacted normally to chronic trauma and disrupted attachment, I would not have developed DID. Trauma tried to tell me that I was not human and that I should be excluded from humanity. An overemphasis on parts blotted out the other equally significant impacts of trauma such as somatisation and the difficulties we have with ascribing realistic meaning to our circumstances.

Making us out to be 'special', even if positively intended, making us the subject of TV documentaries for people to ogle at, can have the effect of further separating us from the normal spectrum of humanity. And it can blend dangerously with our innate, traumagenic sense of worthlessness and shame, to offer us an identity in being 'special' that can bring with it at least some attention. It may be negative attention, in terms of stigma and discrimination and the unutterable attacks of some DID-denying internet 'trolls', but often any attention is better than none. But this can just perpetuate the cycle of psychological and emotional abuse in our lives. We do not resist it, because we have become conditioned to accepting that we are not really human and that we do not really have any rights, and that this is the way that it ought to be. Better to poke us with a stick than ignore us altogether.

But I have come to believe very strongly indeed that I am not special, that I am not weird, and as a result I do not want to show myself off in a sensationalist way. I am a normal person who has responded in normal ways to some abnormal treatment: DID is no more exceptional than the colour of our skin having adapted over long periods of time to environmental exposure to the sun.

I have been helped enormously by working with a therapist who does not gawp at my multiplicity but who demands growth and forward movement from me every single week. 'DID is not an excuse for bad behaviour,' she told me at an early point. Or self-centeredness or egotism or laziness or cowardice, all of which lie latent within me. She views me as a human being just like her. She does not patronise me, or treat me as if I am 'special'. She does not relegate me to some sub-human category of being, or deride me with a label. She welcomes each of my parts, and there is not the least flinching surprise when any of them appear in our session together. But they appear for us to continue our work, at the frontier edges of my psyche, labouring to try to integrate all of me into some connected 'whole'—my parts, my experiences, my feelings, my memories, my body, my thoughts, my attachments, my beliefs, my boundaries, my perceptions, my shame and all the unhealed suffering that seems to go on forever deep within me. Sometimes I need dissociation still to cope with it, but slowly that need is ebbing away, and slowly a more complete version of 'me', the sum of all my parts, is emerging.

I see it as the mental equivalent of joined-up writing: none of the letters lose their significance, their meaning or their existence. But they all begin to join together to form words and sentences and prose, which carries a greater impact than any single letter or digit on its own. The parts of the personality form together to create a unified, meaningful whole.

And I, and all my parts, want to write some great prose with my life. Parts are not the problem: parts coming together are the solution.

Dissociative Moments

I am sitting at my desk, alone. But I don't feel alone. Everything is normal, but everything is different. There are sounds from the birds scrabbling on the roof. They are two metres above me, by the skylight. But they are far, far away. The walls are a pale yellow but their vibrancy seems to grab me. My eyes are sucking in their colour. I am falling back, deep down into myself. I am fuzzed in a fog. I am outside myself and deep within myself all at the same time. I am having a dissociative moment.

Moments like this happen all the time. Sometimes I know what has triggered them; at other times, it's a complete mystery. I feel myself floating. I feel as if everything around me has become unreal. I feel that I, myself, am unreal. Things that are familiar become unfamiliar. Characteristics, such as colours, or shapes, or the contrast of light against the dark, stand out and grab my attention as if I am looking through a tube at them: everything else fades away, and there is just this one thing, this one mostly irrelevant thing, this life-hanging-on-it one thing and I can't feel anything else or see anything else or do anything else but have my attention consumed by it.

Dissociative moments, falling into the mental fog, detaching from the body…And I don't always know what happens next. Sometimes it just dissolves and I'm back again, bewildered a little, feeling wrung-out, like I'm scrabbling around on the inside to hang onto myself. I feel mentally dizzy, disoriented, like I've just stepped off a kids' roundabout. And always, always, the instinctive need to act normal, to try to make sure that no-one has seen. The fear isn't that I dissociated; the fear is that someone noticed.

At other times I can't or I don't pull back from the brink, and I disappear inside. If I'm aware of it, it's like falling into sleep or an anaesthetic. Sometimes, when I'm inside, deep, deep down inside myself, I can see what's happening still on the surface. But I'm watching it from afar, and it's not me I'm watching. This is co-consciousness, the strangest feeling in the world. I can see myself talking and interacting and doing and feeling, and yet it's not myself, it's just someone else, someone I don't know, someone I have no connection with.

What they do and what they say surprises me. I don't know what's coming next. It just is. It just happens. Sometimes I hear my mouth saying things and, with thoughts crawling as if through glue, I think, deep inside, No! Why are they saying that? What's going on? If it's too much then my thoughts just squash up into themselves and stop altogether and there's blank.

When I'm gone completely—when I've switched to another part and I–as–me has lost contact altogether—then I only have the report of others to go on. That's when you see the most obvious signs of dissociative identity disorder—an adult shifting perceptibly in the way we talk and hold our body and shift our eyes and interact with the world, until there is something so much evidently younger about us, or different in some other striking way: the angry, hostile side of us that you've never seen before; the emotion-spurting adolescent; the ragged, raw, empty child-me.

But me as adult-me: what do I know of my other selves? Six years ago, nothing. When I switched, I switched completely. I was gone, and nothing of what else I was in my other selves came through. Afterwards, when I was back, there was just a bustle of noise and prickly emotion in my head, all of it incomprehensible, like I had someone else's feelings and I didn't even know what they were. I relied on my husband or my therapist to tell me what I had been. They would describe the characteristics of my switch: a younger presentation of myself, traumatic memories blurting out in anguished distress, these parts all consumed in defending against some over-real threat. My husband or therapist would describe it to me, and I listened and accepted what they were saying as true, but in a detached, uninvolved way, as if they were recounting the plot of a film. It wasn't me they were describing. It wasn't relevant. It was curious, maybe embarrassing, but that was all. And too much information from them, too accurate a rendering of what I had been like, in a way that stirred a connection with what was deep inside me, and I would faze out again: this stuff was dissociated, disconnected and set apart for a reason, and the reason was because it was too painful, too conflictual, for me to know it. So they learned to tell me only slivers and were shocked by my insensitive, crass jocularity. Rob: 'A moment ago you were distraught, and now you're… laughing?' I would shrug my shoulders because the distress was just an ominous discomfort inside, like psychological indigestion, and my laughter was an attempt to swallow it again.

Trauma intrudes continually. Not as much as it used to, now it has an outlet, but for years I didn't even know that trauma was its name. I walk down the High Street and suddenly pain spins up inside me like a corkscrew. I don't know why. I don't know what it is. Then nausea spurts up like a geyser. I'm dizzy, and suddenly everything around me feels unreal, all these people walking along in their unobtrusive uncompanionable anonymity. They are unreal. I am unreal. Pain, nausea, and jarring echoes in my mind of something. A voice, deep inside me, that feels not-me but I know that it's not outside me: Don't hurt me, don't hurt me. And I realise that ten paces behind, a moment ago, was a man with a camera, and I can feel the fear inside, the wailing, the reluctant recoiling of a child part inside of me who was triggered by the man who walked past. A few more steps forwards, and it's past and I breathe again and I whisper inside to myself, It's okay now, it's okay and I remember to breathe and to zoom in on that breathing, in, out, slowly now, in, out, it's okay. And it passes and I'm at the Post Office and I'm back to adult, non-trauma life, back to the life that consists of a hundred of those intrusions every day. I can hold the hand of the little one inside me and I don't switch, I don't lose touch with my surroundings, I just hear the hurt and feel the pain and the nausea, for a moment, a long long moment sometimes, but then it is gone.

I used to think I was mad. Those jarring intrusions, those ego-alien, time-travelling contusions that exploded in my body and mind. What was going on? What were these voices in my head, this crying, this wailing, this screaming, this sobbing? How could I one moment be pleasantly bobbing along and the very next I am a blur of unabridged distress? These thoughts—where did they come from? These feelings? These urges, that aren't my urges? These compulsions? These random, illogical needs? They feel as if they are not coming from me, as if they don't belong to me. Am I mad? No,

I'm not mad: I'm traumatised. This is what trauma does to you—separating you off from yourself, from your experiences, from your now-world. A trigger—a reminder in some tiny, inconsequential way in the here-and-now environment—connects you again to that trauma. That's not madness. That's the beginnings of sanity.

Sometimes the triggers are overwhelming and I switch to another part. But mostly they just barge into my consciousness, unwelcome guests dragging with them a house-party of traumatised feelings and knowledge and perceptions. Switching is easy. Intrusions are not. Switching is a release clause, a checking-out when it's all too much; life is much harder with this constant tumult of dissociative voices, but without the escape. It's exhausting. Am I the me who is calm and objective and competent? Or am I the me who is jumpy and hyperalert, barraged by the irritable, paranoid warnings of a traumatised self? To that part of me, everything speaks danger; everything speaks threat. They see the world through a filter of unrepressed hostility. And I can feel that worldview within myself, but it is not my worldview. Trauma has given them that worldview. I was not traumatised, so I don't feel so wary. Both mindsets exist within me simultaneously—that is what 'multiple' means to me.

But I've had six brutal years now of working through the trauma, working on me connecting again to these others parts of myself, working on empathising with myself and having compassion on myself and making connections and a thousand 'Aha!' moments of understanding so that's why I do that—and I have squirmed with the reluctance of accepting that I have parts and parts who have suffered as they have. I've come to understand why the dissociative barriers have been there: conflicts so huge that no mind could hold them all together in one place at one time. I have DID because of those conflicts: for me the central one is *'I am strong and I will survive and it is shameful to be trampled on'* versus the barefaced reality of *'I am weak and I may not survive and I am constantly being trampled on'*. There are others: 'I love them' and 'I hate them'; 'I need them' and 'they hurt me'; 'I like this' and 'I hate this'; 'I have to deal with this' and 'there's no good way to deal with this'.

» Dissociative Moments

But several years on and the barriers have thinned. I am not egg-boxed in any more, sound-proofed and feeling-proofed against the other parts of myself that I had to dissociate from to survive. So now, after switching, when I'm back, there isn't the ink-black void there used to be. Sometimes when I'm gone, I'm there on the back row, watching warily, unable to intervene, unable to know even what I'm going to do next. But there's a link, a connection, a sense that I'm in the same brain-universe, in the same here-now context as this other part of myself. Or even when I'm not, when there's no co-consciousness, there is a sense afterwards like of dreaming: it's there, on the tip of my tongue, on the tip of my mind, the shadowy-surreal sense of what's just gone on. If I strain, I can remember it.

Mostly, though, I don't want to strain; I still don't want to know most of it. It will be painful, and life clamours all around me with the responsibilities of adulthood: I haven't got time, right here, right now, to feel that pain. I haven't got space, right here, right now, with a real-life teenage foster daughter pouting in a real-life my-phone-credit-ran-out strop, right here, right now. There isn't the capacity on the inside of me, with everything pulled taut with trauma and the exhaustion of going there, for me to feel this right now. So I don't look, I don't strain to see into the dreamworld that is my other selves, and I put it on the shelf until later. I've come to appreciate my need to be able to manage 'normal' life, the here-and-now life of work and adult responsibilities and family life, and I appreciate these dissociative barriers that allow me to do that. But I've also been building doorways into the barriers so that I can come and go as I need to.

Sometimes, I don't know and I can't know what has gone on in a switch, but it leaks back to me later, like icemelt in my mind. I call this 'post-consciousness': the knowing afterwards, when there is air in my lungs and looseness in my muscles, when I've got the capacity to know. When I can breathe, I want to know. I want to connect with these other parts of myself, these guardians and recipients of the too-much that I endured as a child. Their pain now is still too-much but it's not spitting any more, like water in hot fat: the temperature has been turned down. There's more control. Not as much as I'd like, not as much as I need, but it's not the emotional chip-pan fire it used to be. The more I've got in touch with my parts, the less they intrude uninvited into daily life. There is a place for my trauma to come out and be heard, and that's in therapy. Six years has taught me that that's a safe place, that it's a big place, with sturdy, strong walls that can absorb my combustion. It hasn't burst into flames with the ferocity of my suffering. And six years has taught me that it will be there next week too, that I can wait that long, that although there might not be enough time next week, there'll be more time the week after that, and we're not going to run out of time in the end. I can have feelings, I can have big, difficult, skin-shredding emotions and they won't destroy me and there is such a thing as soothing. There is a way to calm down. I can feel big feelings because they won't destroy me. They keep trying, but they haven't succeeded. They're not scaring me so much any more.

Life with dissociation isn't easy. But life wouldn't even be without dissociation, so I'm grateful for it. Slowly the links are being made between the different parts of me, and the different parts of my experience. It gets harder, in a way, the less I switch: I am more conscious of what previously was cut off from me. Knowledge, feelings, urges leak through from the inside parts of me. They are not always welcome; they are not always convenient. But they are all part of the bigger experience of me-being-me that I am striving for through therapy. The more I accept my dissociated experi-ences, the less they intrude. But they do still intrude, and a lot of the time now I know about it too. 'Getting better' doesn't always means 'getting easier', at least not to start with. But the alternative is to remain dissociative for the rest of my life, cut off from parts of me that are, intrinsically, me. And that's just not an option.

Pseudogenic, Iatrogenic, Traumagenic?

How do we Know that Dissociative Identity Disorder is Real?

'So I'm curious. On what do you base your belief in DID?'

This was a tweet I received from a fellow twit based in the US a few months ago. The more I use social media, the more I realise how controversial dissociative identity disorder is. For me, after the last five or six years, it is 'normal'. I write about it, I train about it, I read about it and most importantly of all, I live it on a daily basis. So I'm always surprised when I come across the 'DID-deniers', the majority of whom seem to be based in America. If I do a search for 'dissociative identity disorder' on Twitter, on a daily basis I can come across dozens of tweets from people mocking it, making a joke out of it (some of them stupefyingly tasteless, some actually quite amusing), and most of all attacking its credibility as a psychiatric diagnosis and in fact its very existence.

So when someone I have never met tweeted me to say, 'So I'm curious—on what do you base your belief in DID?' it got me thinking. How to answer? How can I take the totality of my life, the first-hand, this-is-it experience I have had over the last few years and construct out of it some argument that would 'prove' that DID exists? The reality is that all of us will believe what we want to believe, and all of us will deny what we want to deny, and if I am responding to sceptics in the hope that I can change their mind, I am wasting my time. What interests me more is thinking about the journey that I myself have been on that has got me to this point of believing that DID is a valid diagnosis and a very real experience not just for me but also for hundreds of people I have come across in the last couple of years.

I had never heard of the terms 'dissociation' or 'dissociative identity disorder' until just a few years ago. I hadn't even come across 'Multiple Personality Disorder' and I first read the book Sybil about three years ago, and watched the film for the first time just a couple of years ago. I hadn't been exposed to any other media representation of DID that I am aware of. Despite my wide reading and education, Gollum and Sméagol are the nearest I had come to it, and certainly no-one was using technical terms to describe them.

One of the arguments against DID is that it is a disorder created by therapy—it is 'iatrogenic'; literally, its origin is in the treatment. So someone may go into hospital for a back operation during which the bowel is ruptured. The ensuing problems with the bowel are 'iatrogenic'—they were caused by the surgery, the treatment itself. And one of the arguments is that DID is caused by the therapist, planting the suggestion that we have 'multiple personalities'. Either consciously in order to please, or at a completely unconscious level, we then develop the symptoms expected of us. This is the argument levelled at Sybil, and Simone Reinders, a neuroscientist involved in studying DID (and who does in fact believe that DID is a valid diagnosis), concedes that Sybil was 'a manufactured iatrogenic case of multiple personalities… Sybil was manufactured through hypnosis, pentothal and a close involvement between subject and therapist' (Reinders, 2008, p. 45). This case has been the subject of the spotlight in recent months as a new book has been published. Written by Debbie Nathan and entitled Sybil Exposed: The Extraordinary Story Behind the Famous Multiple Personality Case (2011), it gives 'proof' that the allegedly true story was fabricated. (I am yet to understand why anyone thinks a true story is true when Hollywood is involved…) But a number of newspapers, magazines and websites have devoted numerous column inches to discuss the book's 'findings' and some have therefore by extension decided that DID does not exist at all as a valid diagnosis.

I stand up in public on a regular basis, I have written numerous articles and a book about DID with more on the way, and yet I got a cold shiver down my spine when I first read about the exposé of Sybil. The thoughts that ran through my head were: Am I making it all up too? Am I a fraud, a fake? Is this all a case of 'false memories' and am I just subconsciously trying to please my therapist? Am I in fact more 'mad' and more 'bad' than I realised?

I know a lot of people with DID, and a lot of them struggle to believe that they have DID. They struggle to believe that they had a traumatic history, and they struggle to believe that the plethora of symptoms which plague their lives on

» Pseudogenic, Iatrogenic, Traumagenic?

a daily basis are anything other than a sign that they are intrinsically 'bad' or hopelessly 'mad'. Many of us with DID hate our diagnosis, are deeply ashamed of it, and as a result don't want anyone else to know about it. When people start writing articles in newspapers, magazines and blogs claiming that DID doesn't even exist, it is deeply distressing to us. On the one hand, we would like nothing more than to discover that we don't have DID after all—that we don't have multiple personalities; that we don't have a horrific history of childhood trauma or neglect; that we don't have fundamental divisions in our psyche between 'Apparently Normal Personalities' and 'Emotional Personalities' (van der Hart et al, 2006). On the other hand, we would be terrified: if this label, weird and incomprehensible though at times it is, doesn't describe what is going on for us in our daily lives, what on earth is wrong with us? And if we just think we have parts or alters (or whatever other term we prefer to use), when actually they aren't real and they have just been created by the therapist who was supposed to be helping us…then what hope is there for recovery for us, when we are suffering from a non-existent disorder, and the people who are supposed to be helping are actually the ones causing the problem in the first place?

Of course, there is some false logic in the argument that just because Sybil was 'a manufactured iatrogenic case of multiple personalities' (Reinders, 2008, p. 45)—and let's face it, just because a journalist says that it was, doesn't make it so—it doesn't mean that genuine DID doesn't exist. Sometimes in our black-and-white, 'splitting' mentality, we strive to adopt a position that is 'totally true' or 'totally false'. There are some people who experience pseudo-pregnancies and tell people because of their own emotional needs that they are having a baby when they are not. Just because this is the case doesn't mean to say that pregnancy does not exist. The evidence for that is a little bit obvious. So I'm not particularly fussed about whether the case of Sybil is proved to be 'true' or 'false'. Some may argue that it is a public relations disaster for DID, but I don't think it is. I actually think that the further away we can move from a stereotype of multiplicity, and the model of Sybil as a kind of 'gold standard' for DID, the better it will be for all of us. There is no doubt that Sybil—the book, but especially the film—brought Multiple Personality Disorder into public consciousness. But there is also an argument that it provided a skewed representation of what dissociative identity disorder actually is—a caricature that it is very difficult for us all now to get away from.

So, firstly then, is DID real? The iatrogenic argument for DID, also know as the sociocognitive model, is that either at a conscious or an unconscious level, the dissociative phenomena such as 'multiple parts of the personality' are created, or encouraged, or exaggerated as a result of expectations from the therapist. Where this argument immediately falls down in my case is that I had dissociative symptoms many, many years before I first sat in a therapist's room.

I had what I would term my first 'breakdown' during my second year at University. For several weeks I was found at various times by various friends in College wandering around vaguely in the middle of the night, staring into space or rocking, and acting and speaking in a childlike manner. They reported that I was 'not myself', that I seemed to be afraid of 'the men coming', that I didn't like 'the ropes' and so on. I had absolutely no motivation whatsoever to do this for attention or secondary gain at the time—it remains one of the most painfully embarrassing and shameful times of my life. I was at Cambridge University, a high-flying student with significant academic potential, and I was 'acting mad' and in a way that just resulted in me being ostracised from my peer group and brought me to the stern and unforgiving attention of the College tutors, whose 'pastoral care' of me had as its only goal my achieving a First. I was mortified at what was reported back to me about what had taken place during these episodes of 'lost time'. I would have done anything to stop them happening and for me not to suffer the loss of respect and reputation that resulted in that most demanding of environments.

After I left College a couple of years later, again I suffered a kind of 'breakdown' during which suicidality and self-harm were once more high on the agenda. Friends would report 'strange behaviour', especially that which would appear to be from a much younger part of me, accompanied by inconsolable terror and accounts of horrific abuse. I did my best to hide it all. I didn't want anyone to know. I was shamefully afraid that I was 'insane' and that if I went to a GP about it, I would be admitted to a psychiatric ward and never let out again. I feared for my job, my career, my ability ever to form a relationship or marry or have kids. I didn't want anyone to know, so my bizarre behaviours were kept to a couple of discreet friends, one of whom was my housemate and from whom it was impossible to hide quite so much 'insanity'.

It was over ten years later before I began to have counselling. By then, in 2005, I had suffered a catastrophic breakdown which affected every area of my life, and for nearly a year I teetered on the edge of existence, trying to cope with life by day whilst at night a whole series of 'alter personalities' or 'parts' made themselves known to my husband and one close friend. Again, we hid everything. I didn't want anyone to know. I was deeply ashamed. I wouldn't even see the GP about 'normal' stuff, in case she somehow figured out what else was going on. My husband met parts of me called 'Diddy', who was 4 years old, and 'Charlie' who was an 8-year-old boy, and 'Switch', who was again male and about 12. And then, eventually, at the end of ourselves, after 13 months of chaos and not being able to keep it hidden any longer, I started counselling.

But I entered therapy with the express intention of not 'dissociating'. I don't know where I had picked the word up from. I had read a lot of books to try to make sense of what I was experiencing, and was shocked to realise that the flashbacks of abuse I was experiencing, the guilt, the shame, the self-harm, the anger, the insomnia, the physical pain, the edginess, the hypervigilance, the startle reflex, the panic, the confusion—all of it was 'normal'. The nearest I could get to an accurate label was 'post-traumatic stress disorder'.

But somehow, somewhere, the word 'dissociation' played a role even though I didn't know what it was. I went into counselling very much determined not to mention the fact that I had these little episodes of lost time, during which my husband dealt with a child part hiding under the table who didn't want her wrists to be tied any more. I wanted this counsellor to help me, not think I was mad and untreatable. I fully intended to be thoroughly normal while I was in counselling so that I could get better quickly and quietly.

It took about three months for 'parts', or 'alters' to appear in counselling. I was mortified to realise that I didn't know what had gone on for most of the session that day. Perhaps it was because we'd had to use a different room. I don't know what triggered it, but I did have towards the end of the session that familiar sense of waking up from a deep dream and not being able to quite remember what we had just been talking about. In private, I berated myself, lectured myself in a 'must do better' kind of a way, and hoped against all hope that I hadn't messed the whole thing up by acting 'weird'. It was the Summer months anyway and so sessions were a little more ad hoc than they had been up to that point. I was relieved, because it gave me a break to pull myself together and make sure that I didn't 'lose time' again.

I'm not sure what happened next but I do know that 'lost time' became a feature of our sessions and that it became a kind of talked-about-but-not-talked-about thing. It just seemed a natural and logical extension of what had gone on in our earlier sessions, where I had watched myself talking but from a distance and wondered what on earth I was going to say next, because I had no idea. I had listened to myself talk about a rape in a stables, and I really and literally didn't know what happened next—until I said it. Then I would go home and beat myself up for lying and making it all up, and yet with a deeply anxious sense that I wasn't, and that it was true, and that I knew it was. But on an emotional level it was certainly easier to believe that I was just making it all up.

A few months went by and the puzzle of what I was, the puzzle of what my behaviour meant, was getting bigger as my behaviour became more bizarre and I lost more and more time during sessions. My husband was used to it at home, and we look back now and wonder why we never really tried to figure out what was going on. It just

» Pseudogenic, Iatrogenic, Traumagenic?

was. It didn't really occur to either of us that there might be a name for it, a label to describe it, and that it was something that other people did too. I think I just assumed that it was part of my inherent 'badness' and that I needed to keep on trying, and maybe a bit harder, to 'stop it'.

And then one day in my session, towards the end, my therapist produced a booklet about trauma and dissociation, and suggested I read it. I took it away and devoured it instantly, and there was that awful, stomach-sinking feeling that I was reading something that described me. Suddenly 'it'—'it' being the madness of my behaviour—had a name: 'dissociative identity disorder'. I sat and tried to argue with it, pointing out all the ways that I wasn't an exact match and that it didn't really apply to me, but at the beginning of my next session, we talked about it together. 'Is this—me?' I asked. 'What do you think?' came back the reply. 'Is this what I've got?' And again: 'What do you think?' I shrugged. 'Maybe.' I hoped: 'Maybe not.'

A few months later I started to see a new therapist. This new one had lots of experience working with DID. I decided to play it cool, try to get her to realise that I wasn't mad, that I was just a normal member of society, just like her. But by the end of the first assessment session, to my horror, fourteen of my alters had introduced themselves to her. I came back into the room with that foggy sense of having been somewhere but I couldn't quite remember where, just like in a dream. 'Do you think I've got DID?' I asked. I was desperately hoping that she would say no, because then I wouldn't have a label, I wouldn't have this 'thing' hung around my neck like a millstone that marked me apart from 'normal' people and placed me on the 'other side of the table' as I saw it at the time. In my professional career, I had always been on the 'right' side of the table, and I had seen the way that people on the 'other side' were treated and referred to, especially when they weren't there. I never ever wanted to be on the 'other side', and yet by having a label, having a psychiatric diagnosis, I knew that I would be—and I hated it.

'Oh yes,' the therapist replied breezily, 'absolutely no doubt about it at all.' And she seemed so nonchalant about it, as if I'd asked her if I had brown hair, that somehow some of the shame receded, but I still recoiled inside with that awful sense that I couldn't get away from facing that reality any more.

According to the iatrogenic model, I shouldn't have had any 'parts' or 'alters' until I started therapy. But they were there over ten years previously, at College, and afterwards when I left and shared a house with a friend. They were there for a whole year, my annus horribilis of breakdown and utter insanity, before I entered therapy for the first time. My first therapist, for nearly a year, observed what was happening and eventually, tentatively, suggested a label that seemed to fit. But she wouldn't be definitive about it. It was left to me to decide that the glove fitted. It was a glove that, if I'd wanted to, I could have thrown away, and I could have just kept talking about suffering from a 'breakdown' or even 'post-traumatic stress disorder'.

I eventually completed some screening tools and when I was discussing the results of them with my GP she started tapping away on her computer. 'How do you spell it?' she asked, and dutifully typed in what I told her. I sort of wanted something more official than that, but I was also mortified at even that brief description appearing on my medical records. I have since found out that it's best not to volunteer mental health information if you ever want to get reasonably-priced life insurance.

The case of Sybil suggests that iatrogenic DID is a possibility. I am equally convinced that in my case, and in the case of many people that I know, that is not what has happened. I believe that my DID is traumagenic, that is to say that it was caused by early, chronic, extreme abuse, which occurred on an existing fault-line of disorganised attachment.

But I do also believe that we can be consciously or unconsciously 'encouraged' to present in a more dramatic way than we need to. We can feel the pressure to 'fit in', to be 'proper DID' and behave accordingly. This is a fear that many professionals have, and sometimes rightly so, about what happens when dissociative survivors meet together. Will we 'encourage' one another to 'act out', will we simulate each other's symptoms, and imitate what we 'should' be like—for example, by pretending to switch to a younger alter or exaggerating a switch or childlike behaviour? I think that on occasions this happens. After all, it happens in all groups in order to fit in. The same can be true of dissociative groups. But it can be true in a positive sense as well, in that if what is modelled is good coping strategies, control over switching, taking responsibility for ourselves and appropriate relating, then that can have a positive impact and empower dissociative survivors to cope well with their symptoms too.

I think the vast majority of people with DID that I have met are genuinely dissociative. Most of us worry that we have 'made it all up', especially when we are co-conscious. It's hard to believe that what you are saying is true when you 'hear' yourself saying it from a distance and at the very same moment you're thinking, 'But I didn't know that.' The experience of co-consciousness, of having two separate and distinct but co-existing streams of consciousness, is a very strange concept and not one that is easy to explain to people who do not experience it. I have met many, many people who fear that they are simulating DID because they 'observe' themselves as separate parts of the personality. Often what happens is that, because we are so averse to the dissociative diagnosis and so phobic of the realities of the abuse that led to that dissociation, we often declare to ourselves and especially to our therapists that, 'We're not really DID after all—we're making it all up.' This is one of the arguments used to 'prove' that Sybil was making it all up—because she said so. I don't know the truth in that particular case but it did make me smile: it's a self-directed accusation I hear on a very regular basis from many genuine DID people. If only we could convince people (ourselves included) that we are normal!

But I do also believe that there are cases of 'false' DID. Some of the literature on this subject (Reinders, 2008; Brand et al, 2006) divide DID cases into traumagenic (i.e. genuine), iatrogenic (caused by the therapy) or pseudogenic (falsified). There is a certain amount of research and debate around the issue of pseudogenic diagnoses, and most people divide it into two types. Firstly there is malingering, which is where symptoms are feigned for financial, legal or other gain, including exculpation for crimes. And secondly there is 'factitious' presentation, where the person feigns symptoms not for financial reasons, but in order to assume the sick role, to meet personal or emotional needs, or to avoid responsibility. This can be at either a conscious or unconscious level.

Rogers (1997) estimated that 7-17% of psychiatric diagnoses are malingered. As far as factitious psychiatric diagnoses are concerned, that rate is between 0.5% and 6%. Factitious presentation of dissociative disorders are between 2% and 14% according to Brand et al (2006). So the research literature clearly points to the fact that some cases of mental health diagnoses, including dissociative disorders and DID, are clearly 'false'. However, Nijenhuis and van der Hart make an interesting point that 'these problems of malingering, factitious disorders, and simulation are not at all unique to or heightened in DID but occur with similar frequency in other genuine mental disorders' (Nijenhuis & van der Hart 2009, p. 467). So, yes there is such a thing as 'fake DID' but no more than people feigning other disorders.

Again with our black-and-white need to split, within the DID world we want to believe that everyone we meet who claims to have DID is real DID, not factitious or malingered, but clearly a percentage are subconsciously or consciously making it up. Those of us with trauma backgrounds generally struggle enough with suspicion, paranoia and mistrust as it is, so to figure that maybe around 10% of people we meet who claim to have DID may not actually do so is worrying. So can we tell the real cases from the fake ones?

A research study by Coons & Milstein in 1994 was based on 112 consecutive admissions to a dissociative disorders unit and they found that 10% of them had factitious or malingered DID. So how did they distinguish the real from the fake? 'An exaggerated, highly dramatic clinical presentation, combined with classic symptoms of malingering characterised the malingered or factitious DID cases...Malingerers often had a history of lying, made claims of fantastic and

» Pseudogenic, Iatrogenic, Traumagenic?

unbelievable psychological symptoms, and refused to allow information to be obtained from collateral sources' (Brand et al, 2006, p. 66). So people who are faking it are often a bit over-the-top about it—they exaggerate. One study (Welburn et al, 2003) also showed that genuine DID patients showed more signs of distress and dissociation during the assessment interviews than those faking it. Draijer & Boon (1999) point out in their study that they were able to distinguish between genuine and simulated DID because real DID people evidenced higher levels of anxiety, more shame and more conflict over their diagnosis. This very much fits with my experience of DID—it's not something that most of us want to shout from the rooftops and it's not something that we find easy to talk about. The majority of people I know are highly conflicted about admitting to having DID and although I am nowadays very public about my experience, that wasn't an easy place to come to and still has its difficulties. There remain people in my 'normal life' whom I don't want to tell and from whom I still hide.

So is it straightforward then to tell fake cases of DID from real ones? Well, not really, no. Because as Brand goes on to say, 'A small group (less than 10%) of genuine DID patients are reported to present in a dramatic fashion, so this indicator may not be reliable' (Brand et al, 2006, p. 67). In other words, people who are faking DID seem to have extravagant claims to their psychological symptoms, but that is actually part of the experience of being DID as well. It is fantastical—switching between personalities, the abuse we suffered as children, is often so far beyond people's imagination that it seems that it cannot, must not be real. And yet it is. Just because something doesn't seem real doesn't mean that it isn't: just look at the controversy caused by the revelation that the earth is round.

The other issue that I think is important is to what extent we may hide our symptoms (going one way down a spectrum), or exaggerate them (going the opposite way up that same spectrum) in order to have our needs met. I am reassured by Kluft's finding that 'only 6% make their DID obvious on an ongoing basis' (2009, p. 600), because this is my experience of living with DID—although I speak publicly about having DID, no-one apart from my therapist and my husband sees my 'parts'. None of my friends, none of my colleagues, none of the people in my locality see any evidence of me being dissociative, unless there is a 'perfect storm' of circumstances and I've failed to take notice of the signs that I am heading out of my window of tolerance and it has got to the point of being out of control. Several years ago, that happened fairly regularly but nowadays it is a rare occurrence as I have learned communication and co-operation between the different parts of me. Generally, it's a private thing.

But it's a reality that everyone—people with or without psychiatric conditions—will hide their symptoms if it's adaptive to do so. If we need to be well to do a presentation at work that has repercussions for our career, we are likely to mask our symptoms as much as we can, even if those are only symptoms of a cold. But if we need to make a point to the doctor to get what we need in terms of medication or treatment or referral, we all tend to exaggerate our symptoms. That is normal. And the same thing happens within DID as well. Mostly I would say that we try to hide our symptoms because as Elizabeth Howell says, DID is 'a disorder of hiddenness' (2011), but sometimes some of us will exaggerate our dissociative symptoms in order to get our needs met, and I believe that some of this is behind what people might label as 'iatrogenic DID'. It is not that we do not have DID at all and are pretending (pseudogenic DID, either factitious or malingering). It is that we can feel that there is a certain way to be in order to be 'proper DID', and that can be affected by media representations such as Sybil and more recent publications, or by the role models around us.

So is DID real? Well there is a growing body of research to suggest that you can't fake DID to a neuroscientist. There have been a large number of brain imaging studies using various neuro-imaging techniques, including structural magnetic resonance imaging (sMRI), positron emission tomography (PET scan) and single photon emission computed tomography (SPECT). It is always hard to speculate about the precise brain mechanisms involved due to the wide diversity of neuroimaging techniques used and the methodology and focus of the studies. But there have been four rigorous, larger-scale studies (Vermetten et al, 2006; Reinders et al, 2006, 2008; Sar et al, 2001, 2007) which basically suggest that there are differences in the brains of people with DID compared to others.

For example, Vermetten et al (2006) looked at the volume of the hippocampus and amygdala and found that hippocampal volumes were 19.2% smaller in people with DID, and amygdalar volumes were 31.6% smaller in people with DID compared to those without DID. The researchers think that the hippocampus and amygdala are smaller in DID patients due to trauma and abuse, which supports a traumagenic model of DID.

Reinders et al (2006, 2008) looked at blood flow in the brain and they saw differences between DID people's 'Apparently Normal Personalities' and their 'Emotional Personalities' when listening to a trauma script compared to a neutral script. The ANPs had the same kind of blood flow when listening to both types of script, but there was a difference when the EPs listened to the traumatic material in comparison to the neutral script, suggesting that EPs process or think about traumatic material differently to ANPs. This fits with my experience as an ANP where I can listen to even my own traumatic material and have no emotional reaction to it, as if it were non-traumatic. It's as if the brain when I'm an ANP does not register trauma as traumatic—it's 'dissociated'. It's my EPs who react 'normally' in that sense to traumatic material, responding to it with high anxiety and distress (increased activation in certain parts of my brain). The ANP is actually not 'normal' because they are not distressed by distressing material. That's why we can continue with normal life as if this stuff isn't going on for us, totally switched off from it.

But all the science in the world won't convince people—just think global warming nowadays or the dangers of cigarette smoking in the 1960s. At the end of the day I am convinced that DID is real because it is part of my day-to-day existence. I am reassured that there are some scientific studies emerging that validate my experience, as well as hypotheses such as the theory of structural dissociation (van der Hart et al, 2006). I believe that certain cases of DID can be iatrogenic. And I also believe that it can be pseudogenic—either factitious (for emotional gain, often unconsciously), or malingered (for financial or other gain, often consciously).

But just because some people make it up, consciously or otherwise, doesn't mean to say that it doesn't exist, just like the analogy of pseudopregnancy. If we could get away from the Sybil stereotypes, it might help, but the sad thing is that we suffered disbelief and denial as children and this is re-enacted for us in so many contexts again as adults. It is distressing enough to suffer from DID as it is, without the added weight of people not believing that it even exists. I am reassured that rates for 'false' DID are no higher than for any other psychiatric diagnosis. I am also reassured that there are bodies such as the ISSTD and ESTD (European Society for Trauma and Dissociation) and that they have produced guidelines for treating DID—there are lots of people who take this condition seriously nowadays. But perhaps, as I say on training days, 'denial of the syndrome is part of the syndrome', and so the hardest battle is for us to believe it ourselves.

The Problem of Prevalence

by Karen Johnson

On Pages 23-24 we provide a table of statistics detailing the prevalence rates for dissociative identity disorder and other dissociative disorders based on a number of studies conducted across the world. Statistics like these are not merely academic. They tap into fundamental questions that haunt many of us survivors: Am I the only one? Am I all alone? Many therapists ask the questions: is DID rare, and is it therefore something I am unlikely to come across in my professional career? Because if it is rare, perhaps I don't need to know about it, and certainly I don't need to spend time and money on training for it. Or if I do happen to come across DID, is it so specialist (another word, really, for rare) that I should immediately refer it on? Or is DID, as the ISSTD (International Society for the Study of Trauma and Dissociation) believe, 'relatively common' (2011, p.118)?

As a survivor with DID, it makes a big difference to me whether DID is common or rare. Are there other people like me? Are there enough people with DID in this country for it to warrant research and NICE treatment guidelines? Or am I all alone in this, unlikely to meet anyone else who can empathise with my experience? Is it just me? Some people might relish the thought of being that unique or 'special', but personally I would prefer to feel less alone. I don't want to be 'rare'. I don't want to be sensationalised. I don't want a therapist, or anyone else for that matter, to recoil with shock at meeting someone with DID as if an almost-extinct Javan Rhino has just sat down on the chair opposite them. Whilst I don't really want to be labelled (I'll save my ambivalence about that for another article!) I do want appropriate understanding and treatment, and most importantly to know that I am not alone.

My experience, of course, through PODS' training days and similar events, is that I now know an awful lot of people with DID and I have a significant group of people I would classify as 'friends' who all have DID too. Anecdotally it doesn't seem rare to me at all. But what does the research say? The research, I have to admit, is a bit ambiguous. The ISSTD in their updated Treatment Guidelines (2011) place the prevalence of DID at about 1-3% of the general population. But studies that these guidelines refer to show that prevalence of DID ranges from 0.4% (Akyüz et al, 1999) to 14% (Sar et al, 2007) and studies of all dissociative disorders range from 1.7% (Akyüz et al, 1991) to 40.8% (Ross et al, 2002). So which is right—less than 2% or over 40%? And how on earth can anyone be certain of the accuracy of these results when we're talking not just about a difference of a few percentage points but massive discrepancies?

Understanding statistics is hard enough as it is, without the facts being buried in obscure research papers. Newspapers are forever quoting seemingly-random percentages for all manner of 'scientific studies' that tell us that we need to exercise twenty minutes a day, or an hour a day, eat less than six grammes of salt a day or less than one gramme. We are understandably quite suspicious of facts and figures as mostly we don't understand or know where they have come from—as the joke goes, 90% of statistics are made up.

So where do the figures pertaining to the prevalence of DID and dissociative disorders actually come from, and why do they differ so wildly? The first thing to take into account is whether the study is based on inpatients, outpatients or people in the general community. This can made a big difference: you would expect to see a higher rate of mental health disorders on an inpatient unit than you would in the general population, despite that other joke about how people who work on mental health units are more mad than their patients...

A review of prevalence studies shows that DID is found in 0.4% to 7.5% of psychiatric inpatients (Sar, 2011). Rates for outpatients—so people accessing mental health services but on an appointment basis—range from 2% to 6% for DID. And finally, community studies—so research based on people with no involvement with mental health services, i.e. 'Joe Bloggs'—show the prevalence of DID ranging between 0.4% and 3.1%. That would equate to quite a large number: between about 250,000 to just under two million people in the UK. To put that in perspective, prevalence rates for schizophrenia generally sit around the 0.55-1% range of the general population (Goldner et al, 2002). So arguably more people have DID than schizophrenia and yet rigorous research, appropriate treatment services, charity support and government investment for schizophrenia far outstrip anything available for people with DID.

But DID is only the top end of the spectrum. When researchers look at the whole range of dissociative disorders, prevalence varies between 4.3% and 40.8% in inpatient samples (Sar, 2011), 12% to 38% for outpatient samples (Brand et al, 2009a) and 1.7% to 18.3% for community samples (Sar, 2011). So in theory between roughly 1 million and 11 million people in the general UK population suffer from a dissociative disorder of some description. That is an awful lot of people, and it's a huge variation.

In order to make sense of such differing rates, it is vital to consider what it is that prevalence studies are looking for. There has to be a definition of the disorder that they are seeking to study. So how do you define DID, and how do you define dissociative disorders? Do you take the diagnostic criteria of the DSM-IV (Diagnostic and Statistical Manual) as the benchmark for what actually constitutes DID? This was updated in May 2013 to the DSM-5, which defines it slightly differently, but I will stick with the DSM-IV criteria, as this is what all the studies in this article are referring to. The DSM-IV defines DID as:

- The presence of two or more distinct personality states, each with its own relatively enduring pattern of perceiving, relating to, and thinking about the environment and self.

- At least two of these identities or personality states recurrently take control of the person's behaviour.

- Inability to recall important personal information that is too extensive to be explained by ordinary forgetfulness.

- The disturbance is not due to the direct physical effects of a substance (e.g. blackouts or chaotic behaviour during alcohol intoxication) or a general medical condition (e.g. complex partial seizures) (APA, 2000).

Or do you take a different definition, for example the European classification system, the ICD-10 (WHO, 2010)? Or Dell's (2006) more subjective, symptom-orientated model? Or clinical opinion? Variation between studies comes not only from varying diagnostic criteria for DID, but also from the differences in the way that researchers actually measure whether someone meets those criteria. There are a number of screening instruments and interview schedules that researchers use—these include the DES (Dissociative Experiences Scale), the SCID-D-R (Structural Clinical Interview for DSM-IV Dissociative Disorders) and the DDIS (Dissociative Disorders Interview Schedule). To narrow down participants for a study, researchers often first use the DES, which is a self-report questionnaire, and then only include those people with a score higher than the 'cut-off' point of 30. But other researchers use a cut-off level of 20 or even sometimes less. So there is no standardised agreement on the baseline for who is used for the study.

Then there are cultural issues for research samples. As the ISSTD (2011) points out, contrary to accusations from people in the 'DID-denying' camp, DID is not a Western phenomenon and prevalence studies have been carried out in a range of countries and cultures including Saudi Arabia, Turkey, Ethiopia and Uganda. However, cultural understanding and beliefs around dissociative experiences may well affect prevalence scores in studies—for example, if 'possession states' are believed to be supernatural in nature rather than dissociative, it may affect the prevalence rates for some non-Western cultures.

Finally there are also what are known as 'methodological' issues in research studies, which affect how reliably and seriously the data can be taken—variables such as how many people took part in the study and whether data was gathered by self-report or by interviewing by a trained professional. If you have a small sample size of only 15 people, then the percentages can swing one way or another dramatically if just one person falls on either side of the line. If you bump the figures up to a few hundred, that one person won't have nearly as much of an effect. And if a community sample is taken from a deprived inner

» The Problem of Prevalence

city area, for example, then it may not be truly representative of the 'general population'.

Despite these issues, what many of the prevalence studies on DID and dissociative disorders point to or at least hint at is the fact that DID often goes undiagnosed or misdiagnosed. In one study by Foote et al (2006), 29% of his sample had a dissociative disorder and yet only 5% had been previously diagnosed. Sar et al (2000) also saw this in Turkey where 12% of outpatients qualified for a diagnosis of a dissociative disorder and yet only 1% had received one. (Presumably, when researchers come and do these studies, the people with the budgets to treat people afterwards aren't always jumping for joy.) The ISSTD (2011) suggest that someone can spend between 5 and 12 years in the mental health system before receiving a correct diagnosis, and Brand et al (2009b) suggest that on average people receive 3-4 previous diagnoses before gaining a correct one.

It is well documented that DID is often misdiagnosed as borderline personality disorder, psychosis, schizophrenia or bipolar affective disorder, amongst others. There is also a question in many people's minds about whether these are just straightforward misdiagnoses or whether they are 'co-morbidities'—that is to say, whether people are suffering both from DID and one of these other conditions. In a study by Zittel, Conklin and Westen (2005), it was found that 53% of people diagnosed with borderline personality disorder also qualified for a diagnosis of a dissociative disorder, and 11% of them for full DID.

All of this brings into focus the whole concept of what a diagnosis is anyway, and whether the criteria for one particular label are 'right' and whether there can be any overlap between different conditions. Or is it in fact that these disorders exist on a spectrum and it's more a case of a 'buffet lunch' of symptoms rather than a 'set menu'?

For instance, many of the defining aspects of DID from a phenomenological model (looking at the patient's actual experience) include symptoms such as self-harm, suicidal behaviours, disordered eating and relational issues. All of these share features with other diagnoses, such as PTSD, borderline personality disorder or eating disorders. And of course the flipside is also true, that someone without DID can have 'dissociative' symptoms such as a poor sense of self, memory blanks for aspects of one's autobiography, and feeling 'unreal'.

This is why a bit of a debate raged amongst clinicians and researchers about whether the DSM-IV criteria for DID were adequate: the emphasis was on the observable 'presence of two or more identities'. The debate centred around the fact that it is not always easy to observe these 'two or more identities', or even define what this rather ambiguous phrase means! As Elizabeth Howell (2011) points out, DID is 'a disorder of hiddenness' and Richard Kluft (2009) believes that 94% of people with DID try to hide their dissociative symptoms. This is certainly true of me and many people I know—to have to 'perform' for a psychiatrist and bring out 'parts' or 'alters' in order to get a diagnosis feels not only shaming and degrading, but dangerous too. Why would I let someone I've never met before, or don't trust, see the most vulnerable, hidden parts of me? For most of us, we feel huge shame at having 'parts' and do our best to hide them, letting them 'out' as little as possible, and only then in the safety and privacy of a therapy room or at home. And so many people never received a diagnosis of DID because they refuse to be exposed in this way.

The criteria update in 2013 for DSM-5 seems to have come about as a way of addressing this problem. In these latest criteria, the switching between self-states could be self-reported as well as observed by a clinician. As a result, many people who previously would have been classified with DDNOS (dissociative disorder not otherwise specified) because their parts were not evident in the diagnostic interview would now receive the full diagnosis of DID under DSM-5.

Dell (2006) has proposed a different model of DID which is based on a range of symptoms, rather than the exclusive emphasis on 'two or more identities'. He argues that the DSM 'description of DID is deficient because it omits most of the dissociative phenomena of DID and focuses solely on alter personalities' (Dell, 2006, p.1). He believes that a much broader range of elements should be taken into consideration in diagnosing DID, such as flashbacks, somatoform symptoms, and 'partial intrusions' from others parts of the self, for example hearing voices, or 'made thoughts' or temporary loss or gain of a skill or knowledge.

Of course one of the problems with DID is that we struggle enormously with shame and we don't want to be noticed, diagnosed and measured. On top of this, many of us struggle for years with bizarre behaviours and symptoms which we do our best to hide from the world and so we have no idea at all that we suffer from a 'condition' at all. Usually it is only when things get bad enough for us to suffer a breakdown or other circumstances conspire for us to need to seek help, either medically or in the form of counselling, that we begin to admit—not just to others but also to ourselves—that we may have 'problematic' behaviours and a 'disorder'.

The focus on 'two or more identities' can mean, as the research has said, that it takes us many years to get an appropriate diagnosis. But more accurate diagnostic criteria that take into account our actual experience of living with DID rather than a hangover from Sybil would of course again change the way that prevalence rates of DID and dissociative disorders are measured.

I believe that prevalence rates for dissociative disorders are hugely under-reported, but even current levels are frighteningly high (remember 250,000-2,000,000 people in the UK with DID). We do need a better definition of it. We do need more thorough research into accurate prevalence rates. We do need much more 'label awareness' if society as a whole is going to take dissociative disorders seriously and fund treatment for them. But neither should we get hung up on labels.

Essentially I want to be heard, shown compassion and empathy, and to be seen as human, as me. Mostly as dissociative survivors we want therapists and counsellors just to get on and work with us as we are in the therapy room, and labels can sometimes get in the way of that. But the encouraging thing is that DID actually has a very good prognosis if treated appropriately (Brand et al, 2009a).

So I am not the only one. I am not alone. I am not rare. Not a Javan Rhino…but as common in the UK in fact as the hedgehog. So yes, therapists, you are likely to come across dissociative disorders and DID in your everyday practice. In fact, understanding of dissociative disorders is essential for everyone. As Vedat Sar (2011, p.6), a leading researcher in this field, says:

'…due to their link to early-life stress in the form of childhood abuse and neglect, better recognition of dissociative disorders would be of historical value for all humanity including global awareness about and prevention of adverse childhood experiences and their lifelong clinical consequences.'

Book List

The PODS website, www.pods-online.org.uk, has a comprehensive book list with links through to Amazon. Please click through to earn us a small percentage commission—at no cost to yourself!

Recovery is my Best Revenge	Carolyn Spring
Coping with Trauma-Related Dissociation	Suzette Boon, Kathy Steele & Onno van der Hart
Rebuilding Shattered Lives: Treating Complex PTSD and Dissociative Disorders	James A Chu
Treating Complex Stress Disorders	Christine Courtois & Julian Ford (editors)
Treatment of Complex Trauma: A Sequenced, Relationship-Based Approach	Christine Courtois & Julian Ford
Fractured	Ruth Dee
Dissociation and the Dissociative Disorders: DSM-V and Beyond	Paul F Dell & John A O'Neil (editors)
Ritual Abuse and Mind Control: The Manipulation of Attachment Needs	Orit Badouk Epstein, Joseph Schwartz & Rachel Wingfield Schwartz (editors)
The Dissociative Identity Disorder Sourcebook	Deborah Bray Haddock
Trauma and Recovery	Judith Lewis Herman
Understanding and Treating Dissociative Identity Disorder: A Relational Approach	Elizabeth Howell
Today I'm Alice	Alice Jamieson
Waking the Tiger: Healing Trauma	Peter Levine
Healing the Unimaginable: Treating Ritual Abuse and Mind Control	Alison Miller
All of Me	Kim Noble
Trauma and the Body	Pat Ogden, Kekuni Minton & Claire Pain
Understanding and Treating Dissociative Identity Disorder	Jo Ringrose
Eight Safe Keys to Trauma Recovery	Babette Rothschild
Forensic Aspects of Dissociative Identity Disorder	Adah Sachs & Graeme Galton (editors)
Mindsight	Daniel Siegel
The Child Survivor: Healing Developmental Trauma and Dissociation	Joyanna Silberg
Feeling Unreal	Daphne Simeon
Attachment, Trauma and Multiplicity: Working with DID (2nd edition)	Valerie Sinason (editor)
Trauma, Dissociation and Multiplicity	Valerie Sinason (editor)
The Stranger in the Mirror	Marlene Steinberg
The Haunted Self	Onno van der Hart, Ellert Nijenhuis & Kathy Steele
First Person Plural	Cameron West
Dissociation in Traumatised Children and Adolescents	Sandra Wieland (editor)

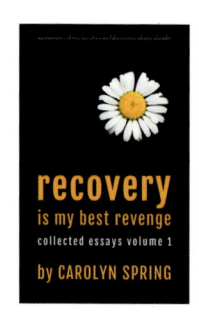

PODS bookstore:
www.pods-online.org.uk/books

Amazon link:
http://tinyurl.com/pods-amazon

Resources

DISSOCIATION » RESOURCE GUIDE » third edition

REFERENCES

Akyüz, G., Dogan, O., Sar, V., Yargic, L. & Tutkun, H (1999). Frequency of Dissociative Identity Disorder in the general population in Turkey. *Comprehensive Psychiatry*. 40(2): 151–159.

American Psychiatric Association. (2000). *Diagnostic and Statistical Manual for Mental Disorders* (4th edition, text revision – DSM-IV-TR). Washington DC: American Psychiatric Press.

American Psychiatric Association. (2013). *Diagnostic and Statistical Manual for Mental Disorders* (5th edition). Arlington, VA: American Psychiatric Publishing.

Baars, E., van der Hart, O., Nijenhuis, E., Chu, J., Glas, G. & Draijer, N. (2011). Predicting Stabilizing Treatment Outcomes for Complex Posttraumatic Stress Disorder and Dissociative Identity Disorder: An Expertise-Based Prognostic Model. *Journal of Trauma & Dissociation*. 12(1): 67-87.

Bernstein, E. & Putnam, F. (1986). Development, reliability and validity of a dissociation scale. *The Journal of Nervous Mental Disease*. 174(12): 727-735.

Boon, S. Steele, K. & van der Hart, O. (2011). *Coping with Trauma-Related Dissociation: Skills Training for Patients and Therapists*. New York: WW Norton & Co, Inc.

Brand, B., McNary, S., Loewenstein, R., Kolos, A. & Barr, S. (2006). Assessment of Genuine and Simulated Dissociative Identity Disorder on the Structured Interview of Reported Symptoms. *Journal of Trauma & Dissociation*. 7(1): 63-85.

Brand, B., Classen, C., Lanius, R., Loewenstein, R., McNary, S., Pain, C., & Putnam, F. (2009a). A naturalistic study of Dissociative Identity Disorder and Dissociative Disorder not otherwise specified patients treated by community clinicians. *Psychological Trauma: Theory, Research, Practice, and Policy*. 1(2): 153-171.

Brand, B., Armstrong, J., Loewenstein, R., & McNary, S. (2009b). Personality Differences on the Rorschach of Dissociative Identity Disorder, Borderline Personality Disorder, and Psychotic Inpatients. *Psychological Trauma: Theory, Research, Practice and Policy*. 1(3): 188-205.

Chu, J. (2011). *Rebuilding Shattered Lives: Treating Complex PTSD and Dissociative Disorders*. New Jersey: John Wiley & Sons, Inc.

Coons, P., & Milstein, V. (1994). Factitious or malingered Multiple Personality Disorder: Eleven cases. *Dissociation*. 7(2): 81-85.

Dell, P. (2006). A New Model of Dissociative Identity Disorder. *Psychiatric Clinics of North America*. 29:1-26.

Dell, P. & O'Neil, J. (Eds.) (2009). *Dissociation and the Dissociative Disorders: DSM-V and beyond*. New York: Routledge.

Draijer, N., & Boon, S. (1999). The imitation of Dissociative Identity Disorder: Patients at risk, therapists at risk. *The Journal of Psychiatry & Law*. 27: 423-458.

Foote, B., Smolin, Y., Kaplan, M., Legatt, M., & Lipschitz, D. (2006). Prevalence of Dissociative Disorders in Psychiatric Outpatients. *American Journal of Psychiatry*. 163 (4): 623-629.

Goldner, E. M., Hsu, L., Waraich, P., & Somers, J. M. (2002). Prevalence and incidence studies of schizophrenic disorders: A systematic review of the literature. *Canadian Journal of Psychiatry*. 47: 833–843.

Haddock, D. (2001). *The Dissociative Identity Disorder Sourcebook*. New York: McGraw-Hill Contemporary.

Howell, E. (2011). *Understanding and treating Dissociative Identity Disorder: A relational approach*. New York: Routledge.

International Society for the Study of Trauma and Dissociation. (2011). Guidelines for treating Dissociative Identity Disorder in adults, third revision. *Journal of Trauma & Dissociation*. 12(2):115-187.

Kluft, R. P. (1992). Discussion: A Specialist's Perspective on Multiple Personality Disorder. *Psychoanalytic Inquiry*. 12: 139-171.

Kluft, R. P. (2009). A clinician's understanding of dissociation: Fragments of an acquaintance. In Dell, P. & O'Neil, J. (Eds.) *Dissociation and the Dissociative Disorders: DSM-V and beyond* (pp. 599–624). New York: Routledge.

Loewenstein, R. (1996). Dissociative amnesia and dissociative fugue. In Michaelson, L. & Ray, W. (Eds.) *Handbook of dissociation: Theoretical, empirical, and clinical perspectives* (pp. 307-336). New York: Plenum.

Main, M., & Hesse, E. (1996). Disorganization and disorientation in infant strange situation behaviour: Phenotypic resemblance to dissociative states? In Michelson, L. & Ray W. (Eds), *Handbook of Dissociation* (pp. 107-138). New York: Plenum Press.

Nathan, D. (2011). *Sybil Exposed: The Extraordinary Story Behind the Famous Multiple Personality Case*. New York: Free Press.

Nijenhuis, E., Van Dyck, R., Spinhoven, P., van der Hart, O., Chatrou, M., Vanderlinden, J. et al. (1999). Somatoform dissociation discriminates between diagnostic categories over and above general psychopathology. *Australian and New Zealand Journal of Psychiatry*. 33:512-520.

Nijenhuis, E. and van der Hart, O. (2009). Dissociative Disorders. In Blaney, P. and Millon, T. (Eds.) *Oxford Handbook of Psychopathology* (2nd ed. pp. 452-481). New York: Oxford University Press.

Pearlman, L, & Saakvitne, K. (1995). *Trauma and the Therapist*. New York: WW Norton & Co, Inc.

Putnam, F. (1989). *The diagnosis and treatment of Multiple Personality Disorder*. New York: Guildford Press.

Reinders, A. (2008) Cross-examining Dissociative Identity Disorder: Neuroimaging and etiology on trial. *Neurocase*. 14(1): 44–53.

Reinders, A., Nijenhuis, E., Quak, J., Korf, J., Haaksma, J., Paans, A., Willemsen, A., & den Boer, J. (2006). Psychobiological characteristics of Dissociative Identity Disorder: A symptom provocation study. *Biological Psychiatry*. 60(7): 730–740.

Rogers, R. (1997). *Clinical Assessment of Malingering and Deception* (2nd ed.). New York: Guilford Press.

Ross, C., Duffy, M. & Ellason, J. (2002). Prevalence, reliability and validity of Dissociative Disorders in an inpatient setting. *Journal of Trauma & Dissociation*. 3(1): 7–17.

Sanderson, C. (2006). *Counselling Adult Survivors of Child Sexual Abuse* (3rd Ed). London: Jessica Kingsley Publishers.

Sar, V. (2011) Epidemiology of Dissociative Disorders: An Overview. *Epidemiology Research International*. p. 1-8

Sar, V., Tutkun, H., Alyanak, B., Bakim, B., & Bara, IM. (2000). Frequency of Dissociative Disorders among psychiatric outpatients in Turkey. *Comprehensive Psychiatry*. 41: 216–222.

Sar, V., Unal, S., Kiziltan, E., Kundaci, T., & Ozturk, E. (2001). HMPAO SPECT study of regional cerebral blood flow in Dissociative Identity Disorder. *Journal of Trauma & Dissociation*. 2(2): 5–25.

Sar, V., Unal, S., & Ozturk, E. (2007). Frontal and occipital perfusion changes in Dissociative Identity Disorder. *Psychiatry Research: Neuroimaging*. 156(3): 217–223.

Spiegel, D., Loewenstein, R., Lewis-Fernández, R., Sar, V., Simeon, D., Vermetten, E., Cardeña, E. & Dell, P. (2011). Dissociative disorders in DSM-5. *Depression and Anxiety*. 28(12): 824-852.

Steinberg, M. (1994). *Structured clinical interview for DSM-IV disorders*. Washington DC: American Psychiatric Press.

van der Hart, O., Nijenhuis, E. R. S., & Steele, K. (2006). *The Haunted Self: Structural Dissociation and the Treatment of Chronic Traumatization*. New York: WW Norton & Co, Inc.

van der Kolk, B. & Fisler, R. (1995). Dissociation & the Fragmentary Nature of Traumatic Memories: Overview & Exploratory Study. *Journal of Traumatic Stress*. 8(4): 505-525.

Vanderlinden, J. (1993). *Dissociative experiences, trauma and hypnosis: research findings & clinical applications in eating disorders*. Delft, The Netherlands: Uitgeverij Eburon.

Vermetten, E., Schmahl, C., Lindner, S., Loewenstein, R. J., & Bremner, J. D. (2006). Hippocampal and amygdalar volumes in Dissociative Identity Disorder. *American Journal of Psychiatry*. 163(4): 630–636.

Welburn, K.R., Fraser, G.A., Jordan, S.A., Cameron, C., Webb, L.M., & Raine, D. (2003). Discriminating Dissociative Identity Disorder from Schizophrenia and feigned dissociation on psychological tests and structured interview. *Journal of Trauma & Dissociation*. 4: 109-130.

World Health Organization. (2010). *The ICD–10 classification of Mental and Behavioural Disorders: Diagnostic Criteria for Research*. Geneva: WHO.

Zittel Conklin, C. & Westen, D. (2005). Borderline Personality Disorder in clinical Practice. *American Journal of Psychiatry*. 162: 867-875.